VETERANS: BENEFITS, ISSUES, POLICIES AND PROGRAMS

VETERANS

BENEFITS, ISSUES, POLICIES, AND PROGRAMS

VOLUME 3

VETERANS: BENEFITS, ISSUES, POLICIES AND PROGRAMS

Additional books in this series can be found on Nova's website under the Series tab.

Additional E-books in this series can be found on Nova's website under the E-book tab.

VETERANS: BENEFITS, ISSUES, POLICIES AND PROGRAMS

VETERANS

BENEFITS, ISSUES, POLICIES, AND PROGRAMS

VOLUME 3

TIMOTHY C. ROBERTS
EDITOR

nova publishers
New York

For permission to use material from this book please contact us:
Telephone 631-231-7269; Fax 631-231-8175
Web Site: http://www.novapublishers.com

Additional color graphics may be available in the e-book version of this book.

Library of Congress Cataloging-in-Publication Data

ISBN: 978-1-63117-046-1
ISSN: 2326-7518

Published by Nova Science Publishers, Inc. † New York

CONTENTS

PREFACE

This book provides an overview of the benefits, issues, policies and programs relating to our military service members. Topics discussed in this issue include health care for rural veterans; further actions needed to collaborate on providing health care to Native American veterans; trends and programs of employment for veterans; the VA vocational rehabilitation and employment program; and includes frequently asked questions on military funeral honors and military cemeteries.

Chapter 1 – The Department of Veterans Affairs (VA) is statutorily required to provide VA-enrolled veterans with access to timely and quality medical care. It does so through the nation's largest integrated health care delivery system. Despite the existence of this system, Congress remains concerned that veterans, in particular rural veterans, may not be able to access VA health services. Among veterans enrolled in VA health care, 41% reside in rural or highly rural areas. Compared to urban veterans, rural veterans have higher prevalence of physical illness, lower health-related quality of life, and greater health care needs. Congress has demonstrated continuing interest in modifying VA delivery of care to expand access for rural veterans. Such interest has been demonstrated through report language, statutory mandates, appropriation of funds, and authorization of demonstration projects. In particular, Congress has encouraged the VA to collaborate with federally qualified health centers (FQHCs)—facilities that receive federal grants and are required to be located in areas where there are few providers, particularly rural areas. The VA is generally a provider—rather than a financer—of health care services; however, the VA has statutory authority to reimburse non-VA providers for services that are not readily available within the VA's integrated health care delivery system. VA facilities may consider contracting with outside providers to provide services to rural veterans. One type of facility that the VA has contracted with in the past are FQHCs. Although FQHCs are one type of facility that the VA can collaborate with, FQHCs may be candidates for VA collaboration because, as a condition of receiving a federal grant, they must meet certain requirements that include providing specific types of services, maintaining certain records, and meeting certain quality standards. These requirements, and the leverage that the federal government may have as a funding source, may facilitate VA-FQHC collaboration to provide care to veterans in rural areas. The report discusses four scenarios under which an FQHC might provide health care services to veterans: (1) without reimbursement from the VA, (2) under the VA's fee basis care program, (3) under a contract for specific services, or (4) as a contractor-operated community-based outpatient clinic (a type of outpatient VA facility). Each of these scenarios is discussed because the scenario used for collaboration affects the considerations that may arise. Some considerations that may arise during attempts to increase VA-FQHC collaboration include the costs of care to an FQHC, the VA, and veterans; the capacity of an FQHC to serve veterans in addition to its existing patients; and the compatibility of the VA and an FQHC in terms of the services available, quality initiatives, accreditation, and use of electronic health records. To address these considerations and encourage VA-FQHC collaboration, there are a number of policy levers that Congress might use. These include oversight, an incentive fund, directed spending, statutory mandates, and watchful waiting. Congress may also consider a combination of these levers. This report discusses considerations that may arise during possible attempts to increase VAFQHC collaboration, and describes policy levers Congress might use to encourage VA-FQHC collaboration. These approaches might also be employed to encourage collaboration between the VA and other types of facilities that may serve rural veterans.

Chapter 2 – Native Americans who have served in the military may be eligible for health care services from both VA and IHS. To enhance health care access and the quality of care provided to Native American veterans, in 2010, these two agencies renewed and revised an MOU designed to improve their coordination and resource sharing related to serving these veterans. GAO was asked to examine how the agencies have implemented the MOU.

This report examines: (1) the extent to which the agencies have established mechanisms through which the MOU can be implemented and monitored; and (2) key challenges the agencies face in implementing the MOU and the progress made in overcoming them. To conduct this work, GAO interviewed VA and IHS officials and reviewed agency documents and reports. GAO also obtained perspectives of tribal communities through attendance at two tribal conferences; interviews with tribal leaders and other tribal members, including veterans; and interviews with other stakeholders, such as health policy experts and consultants.

Chapter 3 – Veterans' employment outcomes in the civilian labor market are an issue of ongoing congressional interest. This report offers introductory data on veterans' performance in the civilian labor market as well as a discussion of veteran-targeted federal programs that provide employment-related benefits and services. According to federal data, the unemployment rate for veterans who served after September 2001 is higher than the unemployment rate for nonveterans. Conversely, the unemployment rate for veterans from prior service periods (a much larger population than post-9/11 veterans) is lower than the nonveteran unemployment rate. The varied demographic factors of each of these populations likely contribute to these variations, though their degree of influence is unclear. There are a number of federal programs to assist veterans in developing job skills and securing civilian employment. Broadly speaking, these programs can be divided into (1) general veterans' programs, (2) programs that target veterans with service-connected disabilities, and (3) competitive grant programs that offer supplemental services but may be limited in scope. General veterans' programs begin with transition programs that are provided to exiting members of the Armed Forces. These transition programs cover a variety of topics including information on identifying occupations that align with military skills and specializations, conducting job searches, applying for employment, and navigating veterans' benefits. One of the most common veterans' benefits is educational funding through the GI Bill. The GI Bill programs typically provide funding for tuition, fees, housing, books and supplies, and other educational costs while the veteran is enrolled. Veterans who are no longer eligible for the GI Bill may receive training benefits through the Veterans Retraining Assistance Program (VRAP). Veterans who are seeking employment without obtaining additional training may receive job search assistance and other services from Local Veterans Employment Representatives (LVER). Veterans who wish to pursue employment in the federal government are assisted by several policies that give them preference in the competitive hiring process or, in some cases, allow them to forego the competitive process and be appointed directly. Veterans who wish to start a small business may receive loans and technical assistance from the Small Business Administration (SBA). Veterans with service-connected disabilities who have obstacles to employment may be assisted by the Vocational Rehabilitation and Employment (VR&E) program. This program provides assistance in identifying an occupation that is consistent with the veterans' skills and interests and providing the services (including educational services) necessary to achieve that outcome. Disabled veterans can also receive assistance from the Disabled Veterans Outreach Program (DVOP), which provides assistance in local labor markets. In addition to these nationwide programs, the federal government also funds competitive grant programs for state, local, and private entities to provide employment-oriented services to veterans. These include the Veterans Workforce Investment Program (VWIP), which may provide training or employment services and Veterans Upward Bound (VUB), which prepares educationally disadvantaged veterans for postsecondary coursework.

Chapter 4 – The IL "track"—one of five tracks within VA's VR&E program—provides a range of benefits to help veterans with service-connected disabilities live independently when employment is not considered feasible at the time they enter the VR&E program. These benefits can include counseling, assistive devices, and other services or equipment. GAO was asked to review issues related to the IL track. This report examines (1) the characteristics of veterans in the IL track, and the types and costs of benefits they were provided; (2) the extent to which their IL plans were completed, and the time it took to complete them; and (3) the extent to which the IL track has been administered appropriately and consistently across regional offices.

To conduct this work, GAO analyzed VA administrative data from fiscal years 2008 to 2011, and reviewed a random, generalizable sample of 182 veterans who entered the IL track in fiscal year 2008. In addition, GAO visited five VA regional offices; interviewed agency officials and staff; and reviewed relevant federal laws, regulations, and agency policies and procedures.

Chapter 5 – This report is written in response to frequently asked questions about military funeral honors and military cemeteries. It provides information on the eligibility criteria, required components of the honor detail, and the funeral ceremony. It also cites legislation that mandates that the Department of Defense (DOD) make military funeral honors available to every eligible veteran upon request.

In: Veterans
Editor: Timothy C. Roberts
ISBN: 978-1-63117-046-1

Chapter 1

HEALTH CARE FOR RURAL VETERANS: THE EXAMPLE OF FEDERALLY QUALIFIED HEALTH CENTERS*

Elayne J. Heisler, Sidath Viranga Panangala and Erin Bagalman

SUMMARY

The Department of Veterans Affairs (VA) is statutorily required to provide VA-enrolled veterans with access to timely and quality medical care. It does so through the nation's largest integrated health care delivery system. Despite the existence of this system, Congress remains concerned that veterans, in particular rural veterans, may not be able to access VA health services. Among veterans enrolled in VA health care, 41% reside in rural or highly rural areas. Compared to urban veterans, rural veterans have higher prevalence of physical illness, lower health-related quality of life, and greater health care needs. Congress has demonstrated continuing interest in modifying VA delivery of care to expand access for rural veterans. Such interest has been demonstrated through report language, statutory mandates, appropriation of funds, and authorization of demonstration projects. In particular, Congress has encouraged the VA to collaborate with federally qualified health centers (FQHCs)—facilities

---

* This is an edited, reformatted and augmented version of a Congressional Research Service publication, CRS Report for Congress R43029, prepared for Members and Committees of Congress, from www.crs.gov, dated April 3, 2013.

that receive federal grants and are required to be located in areas where there are few providers, particularly rural areas.

The VA is generally a provider—rather than a financer—of health care services; however, the VA has statutory authority to reimburse non-VA providers for services that are not readily available within the VA's integrated health care delivery system. VA facilities may consider contracting with outside providers to provide services to rural veterans. One type of facility that the VA has contracted with in the past are FQHCs. Although FQHCs are one type of facility that the VA can collaborate with, FQHCs may be candidates for VA collaboration because, as a condition of receiving a federal grant, they must meet certain requirements that include providing specific types of services, maintaining certain records, and meeting certain quality standards. These requirements, and the leverage that the federal government may have as a funding source, may facilitate VA-FQHC collaboration to provide care to veterans in rural areas. The report discusses four scenarios under which an FQHC might provide health care services to veterans: (1) without reimbursement from the VA, (2) under the VA's fee basis care program, (3) under a contract for specific services, or (4) as a contractor-operated community-based outpatient clinic (a type of outpatient VA facility). Each of these scenarios is discussed because the scenario used for collaboration affects the considerations that may arise.

Some considerations that may arise during attempts to increase VA-FQHC collaboration include the costs of care to an FQHC, the VA, and veterans; the capacity of an FQHC to serve veterans in addition to its existing patients; and the compatibility of the VA and an FQHC in terms of the services available, quality initiatives, accreditation, and use of electronic health records.

To address these considerations and encourage VA-FQHC collaboration, there are a number of policy levers that Congress might use. These include oversight, an incentive fund, directed spending, statutory mandates, and watchful waiting. Congress may also consider a combination of these levers.

This report discusses considerations that may arise during possible attempts to increase VAFQHC collaboration, and describes policy levers Congress might use to encourage VA-FQHC collaboration. These approaches might also be employed to encourage collaboration between the VA and other types of facilities that may serve rural veterans.

INTRODUCTION

The Department of Veterans Affairs (VA) is statutorily required to provide VA-enrolled veterans (see *text box*) with access to timely and quality medical care.[1] It does so through the nation's largest integrated health care delivery system, with more than 150 VA medical centers (VAMCs), 800 community-based outpatient clinics (CBOCs), and a range of other types of facilities (e.g., nursing homes) that provide care to more than 5.5 million patients.[2] Despite this, Congress remains concerned that veterans, in particular rural veterans, may not be able to access VA health services. Among veterans enrolled in VA health care, 41% reside in rural or highly rural areas.[3]

Rural-enrolled veterans share certain characteristics that influence access to and the need for care. Compared to urban veterans, rural veterans have higher prevalence of physical illness, lower health-related quality of life, and greater health care needs.[4] Despite their greater need, rural veterans are less likely than urban veterans to use VA or private sector health care services.[5] The disparity in use of health care may be due in part to longer driving distances to VA medical facilities experienced by many rural veterans, relative to their urban counterparts.[6] VA primary care[7] is available within a 30-minute drive for 91% of urban veterans, 38% of rural veterans, and 22% of highly rural veterans.[8] Fewer than half (49%) of highly rural veterans live within 60 minutes of VA primary care.[9]

VA-Enrolled Veterans

Not all veterans are eligible to enroll in the VA. In general, eligibility for enrollment in VA health care operates through a system of eight priority groups, based on veteran status, presence of service-connected disabilities or exposures, income, and/or other factors, such as status as a former prisoner of war or receipt of a Purple Heart.

Once enrolled in the VA health care system, a veteran remains enrolled and does not have to reapply, even if the veteran's priority group changes (due, for example, to a change in income).Veteran status is established by active-duty status in the U.S. Armed Forces and an honorable discharge or release from active military service. Generally, persons enlisting in one of the armed forces after September 7, 1980, and officers commissioned after October 16, 1981, must have completed two years of active duty or the full period of their initial service obligation to be eligible for VA health care benefits. Servicemembers discharged at any time because of service-connected disabilities are not held to this requirement. Veterans returning from combat operations are eligible to enroll for five years from the date of discharge without having to satisfy a means test or demonstrate a service-connected disability.

A service-connected disability is a disability that was incurred or aggravated in the line of duty in the U.S. Armed Forces (38 U.S.C. §101 (16)). The VA determines whether veterans have service-connected disabilities and, for those with such disabilities, assigns ratings from 0% to 100% based on the severity of the disability (38 C.F.R. §§4.1-4.31). Veterans who are eligible on the basis of exposure include those veterans who may have been exposed to Agent Orange during the Vietnam War or veterans who may have diseases potentially related to service in the Gulf War.

Source: CRS Report R42747, Health Care for Veterans: Answers to Frequently Asked Questions, by Sidath Viranga Panangala and Erin Bagalman.

Note: This report focuses on veterans who are enrolled in VA health care; throughout the report "veteran" refers to VA-enrolled veterans unless otherwise specified.

Congress has demonstrated continuing interest in modifying VA delivery of care to expand access for rural veterans. Such interest has been demonstrated through report language, statutory mandates, appropriation of funds, and authorization of demonstration projects. For example, in a 1999 conference report, Congress "urge[d] the VA to partner with existing [health care facilities] to provide outpatient primary and preventive health care services to area veterans in their home communities."[10] In 2006 Congress established the VA's Office of Rural Health (ORH) to coordinate efforts to improve health care for rural veterans.[11] In 2010 Congress established several demonstration projects that aimed to improve care for rural veterans. [12] In 2011, the VA initiated the Congressionally-mandated pilot project called Project ARCH (Access Received Closer to Home), which provided funding for contracts with outside providers to a variety of health care services to rural veterans.[13] Congress has also repeatedly appropriated funds for activities to improve health care for rural veterans.[14]

This report explores one of these approaches to providing care for VA-enrolled veterans, particularly rural veterans, who do not live near a VA facility: VA collaboration with non-VA facilities. In areas where the veteran population is too small to support a VA facility, the total population may be large enough to support other types of facilities; thus, the VA might collaborate with existing non-VA facilities to provide care for veterans. Federally qualified health centers (FQHCs)—outpatient facilities that provide health care in underserved areas—are presented as an example of entities that might collaborate with the VA.[15] One of four different payment mechanisms may be used in this collaboration and these four scenarios are presented separately. Which of the four mechanisms is used is important for the subsequent discussion of considerations that might arise when the VA and FQHCs are deciding whether to collaborate, as well as for discussing policy levers available to Congress.

The report focuses on FQHCs because they provide outpatient primary care in underserved (often rural) areas; as such, they may be located in areas where rural veterans live and are currently used by veterans. For example, a VA-commissioned study estimated that FQHCs located in the District of Columbia, Maryland, Northern Virginia, and eastern West Virginia served approximately 6,500 veterans in 2009.[16] The VA also has a recent history of contracting with FQHCs and of exploring mechanisms to increase its collaboration with FQHCs; specifically, the aforementioned commissioned report included recommendations to increase collaboration and the VA has 52 contracts with FQHCs for the provision of certain counseling services in rural communities where access to a VA facility is limited. (See *Appendix A.)*

FQHCs may also be candidates for VA collaboration because they currently receive federal grants and therefore must meet certain requirements that include providing specific types of services, maintaining certain records, and meeting certain quality standards. These requirements, and the leverage that the federal government may have as a funding source, may facilitate VA-FQHC collaboration to provide care to veterans in rural areas.[17]

This report focuses on considerations that may affect decisions to collaborate or not. It assumes that readers are familiar with both the VA and FQHCs. Where relevant, background information is included to assist the readers with understanding the consideration discussed. More comprehensive background information on the VA and FQHCs is included in *Appendix B* and *Appendix C*. In addition, readers can access other CRS products that describe the VA health care system and FQHCs in greater depth.[18]

After a discussion of considerations, the report presents some selected policy levers available to Congress should they be interested in encouraging such collaboration.

FQHC Care for Veterans: Four Scenarios

The VA is statutorily required to provide VA-enrolled veterans with access to timely and quality medical care,[19] which may sometimes involve using non-VA providers such as FQHCs. An FQHC might provide health care services to veterans under four scenarios: (1) without reimbursement from the

VA, (2) under the VA's fee basis care program, (3) under a contract for specific services, or (4) as a contractor-operated community-based outpatient clinic (CBOC).Which of these four scenarios is used is relevant for the considerations that will be discussed later in the report (see "Potential Considerations for VA-FQHC Collaboration"). In addition, who is in charge of deciding whether to initiate collaboration and the terms of such collaboration, differs in these scenarios. Specifically, a VA decision to enter into a contract with an FQHC (such as is discussed in scenarios 3 and 4) is determined at the facility level.[20]

Care without VA Reimbursement

An FQHC may provide health care services for veterans without reimbursement from the VA. Every FQHC is required (1) to provide care to all individuals regardless of their ability to pay for services and (2) to collect reimbursements for the cost of these services, either from the patient or from a third party payer.[21] Each FQHC must also establish a fee schedule that takes into account local rates for health care services and the costs that the FQHC incurs providing services. The FQHC is then required to establish a separate discounted fee schedule, which is then further discounted or waived based on a patient's ability to pay. Ability to pay is determined by the patient's income relative to the federal poverty level. The statute requires that individuals with incomes above 200% of the federal poverty level pay full charges, while individuals with incomes at or below 100% of the federal poverty level pay only nominal fees.[22]

Fee Basis Care

The VA may reimburse non-VA providers such as FQHCs for specific authorized health care services rendered to specific veterans on a fee-for-service basis (commonly referred to as Fee Basis Care).[23] This program does not represent a formal collaborative relationship between the VA and a particular FQHC. Fee Basis Care is authorized under the following circumstances: (1) when a clinical service cannot be provided at a VA medical center (VAMC); (2) when a veteran is unable to access VA health care facilities due to geographic inaccessibility; or (3) in emergencies when delays could lead to life-threatening situations.[24]

Although fee basis care may include inpatient care, emergency care, medical transportation, and dental services, it is used predominantly to provide outpatient care.[25] The Fee Basis Care Program Office at the local VAMC pre-authorizes outpatient fee basis care if the care is determined to be appropriate, the veteran is eligible for the program, and an appropriate justification has been provided. Once outpatient fee basis care has been authorized, the veteran selects a provider and receives the service. The non-VA provider (e.g., an FQHC) then sends a claim to the Fee Basis Care Program Office at the authorizing VAMC. After the claim is reviewed and processed, the non-VA provider (e.g., an FQHC) receives payment electronically.[26]

Contracts for Specific Services

The VA has statutory authority to contract with non-VA providers such as FQHCs to deliver health care services to veterans in a specific geographic area or veterans requiring a specific set of services.[27] The VA generally purchases health care services that may not be readily available at VAMCs; examples include radiation therapy, diagnostic radiology, cardiology, cardio-vascular surgery, and orthopedics.[28] Under such a contract, the VA would reimburse the non-VA provider at a negotiated rate. The VA has existing contracts with FQHCs for the provision of readjustment counseling services in rural communities where access to a VA facility is limited. (See *Appendix B.)*

Contractor-Operated Community-Based Outpatient Clinics

The VA may use its contracting authority to establish community-based outpatient clinics (CBOCs) operated by non-VA entities such as FQHCs.[29] In general, such contractor-operated CBOCs are open at least five days a week, for a minimum of 40 hours. The contractor (which may be an FQHC) is required to

- provide staff, facilities, equipment, supplies, and all administrative functions;
- meet both VA standards and The Joint Commission accreditation standards;[30] and
- use the VA's electronic health record to document all patient care.

The VA generally pays contractor-operated CBOCs a monthly fee for each enrolled patient (e.g., each patient in the geographic area of the contractor-operated CBOC); payments for each new enrollee begin during the month of the patient's first visit.[31]

POTENTIAL CONSIDERATIONS FOR VA-FQHC COLLABORATION

This section discusses some considerations that may arise during attempts to increase VA-FQHC collaboration. Considerations include (1) the costs of care to an FQHC, the VA, and veterans; (2) the capacity of an FQHC to serve veterans in addition to its existing patients; and (3) the compatibility of the VA and an FQHC in terms of the availability of services, quality initiatives, accreditation, and use of electronic health records.

In general these considerations are relevant to contracted care from FQHCs or specifically the use of FQHCs as contractor-operated CBOCs, and not to reimbursement of FQHCs under the Fee Basis Care Program. However, with regards to cost, the considerations also include the first scenario discussed above: when a veteran seeks care at an FQHC without VA reimbursement. Throughout this report, FQHCs are used as an example of entities with which the VA might collaborate; therefore, similar considerations may apply to the VA collaborating with facilities other than FQHCs.

Costs to FQHCs, the VA, and VA-Enrolled Veterans

Decisions regarding VA-FQHC collaboration might take into consideration the costs to FQHCs, the VA, and veterans. The potential costs incurred by each of these are discussed briefly below.

Costs to FQHCs

FQHCs may incur costs of caring for veterans (1) under contracts to provide specific services, (2) as contractor-operated CBOCs, or (3) in the absence of any formal collaboration with the VA. The following presents three scenarios under which the FQHC could collaborate with the VA, but might still use its own resources to provide care to veterans. It is not possible to determine which scenario is more likely or more or less favorable to an FQHC.

If the amount paid by the VA to an FQHC under a contract for specific services were not sufficient to cover the costs of services provided to veterans, the collaboration would represent a net loss to the FQHC, impairing its ability to serve its existing patients by depleting its resources. The VA generally reimburses non-VA facilities at the Medicare rate;[32] however, the regulation does not address whether the VA is required to pay the FQHC Medicare payment rate, which is usually higher than the general Medicare payment rate for services provided in other outpatient settings.[33] Despite the higher FQHC Medicare payment rate, the Government Accountability Office (GAO) and the National Association of Community Health Centers (NACHC)—the advocacy organization for FQHCs—found that FQHC Medicare rate is generally not sufficient to cover the FQHC's cost of providing services to Medicare beneficiaries.[34] Whether VA reimbursements to FQHCs would be at the general Medicare outpatient rate or the Medicare FQHC rate is not known; and whether either rate would be sufficient to cover the costs of FQHC services provided to veterans is also not known.

Similarly, if the amount paid by the VA to an FQHC functioning as a contractor-operated CBOC were not sufficient to cover the costs of services provided to veterans, the collaboration would also represent a net loss to the FQHC, impairing its ability to serve its existing patients by depleting its resources. The VA pays contractor-operated CBOCs a per-patient per-month fee. If the patients require a high level of care, the fee may not cover the cost of services. Alternatively, if the patients require only a modest level of care, the fee may be more than sufficient to cover the cost of services.

In the absence of a VA contract, an FQHC might still provide services to veterans as it is required to provide services to all individuals living in a particular geographic area regardless of their ability to pay.[35] In this scenario, the FQHC would charge the individual veteran (in accordance with the FQHC's fee schedule) and seek reimbursement from a third-party payer (e.g., a private health insurer or Medicare) if the veteran had one. Some veterans may meet FQHC requirements for reduced or waived costs; in this case, the FQHC might use other funds (such as the amount it receives through its federal grant) to provide care to veterans.

Costs to the VA

The VA incurs costs of services provided to veterans (1) by FQHCs under a contract for specific services, (2) when FQHCs function as contractor-operated CBOCs, or (3) in the absence of any formal collaboration with FQHCs (i.e., when the VA provides the services directly). Whether the VA reimburses an FQHC (under a contract for specific services) under a fee-for-service arrangement (at the Medicare rate or at another negotiated rate) or pays an FQHC (functioning as a contractor-operated CBOC) a per-patient per-month fee, the cost of contracted care may be greater than the cost of providing the care directly. In the absence of formal collaboration with an FQHC, veterans who live a long distance from VA facilities may forgo routine care, potentially allowing manageable conditions to worsen until more intensive (and generally more expensive) care is required. Predicting which scenario is likely to be most cost-effective for the VA is virtually impossible.

These options may be viewed from the perspective of the agency or from the perspective of individual VISNs and VAMCs. At the agency level, if the VA's congressionally appropriated funds do not increase to accommodate additional contracting, the VA may face a trade-off between funding spent on contracts and funding available to provide services at VA facilities.[36] At the VISN level, because the allocation to the VISN does not increase to accommodate additional contracting, individual VISNs may face trade-offs between funding spent on contracted services and funding available to provide services through VA-operated facilities.[37]

At the VAMC level, if the VISN does not increase the allocation to the VAMC to accommodate additional contracting, the facility may face trade-offs between funding spent on contracted services and funding available to provide services directly. Some Veterans Service Organizations (organizations that advocate on behalf of veterans) have argued that increased contracting would reduce the funds available to provide quality care within the VA health care delivery system.[38]

Costs to VA-Enrolled Veterans

The potential costs to veterans may depend on their cost-sharing obligations within the VA system,[39] their cost-sharing obligations at the FQHC (based on income),[40] and the services they require. Under a collaborative arrangement between the VA and an FQHC, the same cost-sharing requirements would apply to veterans who receive a service included in the standard VA medical benefit regardless of whether they receive their care at the VA or at an FQHC. Veterans who receive FQHC services that are not included in the VA standard medical benefit might be required to pay out of pocket for these services.[41] In the absence of formal VA-FQHC collaboration, veterans might have to pay for services at an FQHC that they could have received at a VA facility for little or no cost.

FQHC Capacity

Depending on the terms of a VA-FQHC contract, an FQHC may be strained to provide care to the veterans and its existing population. FQHCs are required to be located in underserved areas and serve underserved populations, which, by definition, have access to few providers.[42] FQHCs are also required to provide care to all individuals regardless of their ability to pay. These requirements often mean that many FQHCs are operating at capacity. If this is the case, then providing services to additional patients (whether veterans or other patients) might push it beyond its capacity, rendering it unable to provide services to everyone seeking care. In such a situation, it is possible that veterans could displace existing FQHC patients, forcing the existing patients to seek alternative sources of care.[43] The likelihood of this displacement occurring may depend on the terms of the contract between the VA and the FQHC. For example, if the contract were to require that veterans receive preference over other FQHC patients, the displacement would be more likely to occur.

An FQHC's capacity may be partially determined by the availability of a sufficient workforce, and provider shortages may impede an FQHC's ability to expand its treatment capacity in response to a formal collaboration with the VA. FQHCs are required to be located in medically underserved areas that, by definition, have provider shortages.[44] FQHCs also focus on providing types of care with documented provider shortages, such as primary care and behavioral health.[45]

The NACHC estimated that, in 2008, health centers had 1,800 too few primary care providers (physicians, nurse practitioners, and certified nurse midwives).[46] The NACHC further estimated that, by 2015, health centers would have between 15,000 and 19,000 too few primary care providers. Even with additional resources from a VA contract, an FQHC may have difficulty attracting new providers because FQHC compensation is less than compensation available in private practice.[47] For all of these reasons, provider shortages may impede FQHC's ability to collaborate with the VA.

VA-FQHC Compatibility

Collaboration between the VA and FQHCs might require compatibility between the two systems in areas including (but not limited to) services available, quality initiatives, accreditation, and electronic health records. Each of these is discussed briefly below.

Services Available

Services available at an FQHC may not align with the VA standard medical benefit, which all VA-enrolled veterans are eligible to receive.[48] The services available, including whether specialty care is available, vary by facility, both within the VA health care delivery system and across FQHCs. Regulation requires FQHCs to provide primary, preventive, and emergency health services; however, specialty care is optional and available specialty services vary by facility.[49] Given this variation, it is possible that FQHCs that contract with the VA may not provide some of the services that veterans need. Conversely, FQHCs may provide certain services—such as dental services—that the VA does not routinely cover.

Quality Initiatives

VA contracts may impose requirements to join in new VA quality initiatives, which an FQHC may not wish to do. VA agency policy defines the quality standards contractors (including FQHCs) must meet. In compliance with a statutory mandate to undertake a comprehensive program to monitor and evaluate the quality of VA healthcare,[50] the VA engages in initiatives to improve the quality of care delivered to veterans. For example, VA is currently undertaking an initiative to implement a patient-centered medical home model at all VA primary care sites, with the intention of improving healthcare delivery by increasing access, coordination, communication, and continuity of care. Keeping up with these initiatives may be costly or otherwise burdensome to an FQHC or other entity with which the VA may wish to collaborate.

Accreditation

The lack of alignment in accreditation requirements between the VA and FQHCs may impede certain collaboration efforts. The VA requires all contractor-operated CBOCs to meet the accreditation standards of The Joint Commission.[51] In contrast, FQHCs are not required to be accredited by a national accreditation agency; instead, Health Resources and Services Administration (HRSA) encourages FQHCs to be accredited by either the Accreditation Association for Ambulatory Health Care or The Joint Commission.[52]

Electronic Health Records

VA contracting requirements with respect to electronic health records may hinder VA-FQHC collaboration;[53] specifically, the VA requires contractor-operated CBOCs to be able to connect to the VA's electronic health records system. Although statute requires that FQHCs report certain data to HHS, have quality assurance systems in place, and maintain billing systems, there is no requirement for a specific type of system.[54] Thus, the systems in place at FQHCs may not be compatible with VA systems.

An FQHC's ability to connect to the VA's electronic health records system might also be a consideration if the VA were to contract with an FQHC for specific services; the care provided by an FQHC may not be documented in the VA's electronic health record, which may limit coordination and continuity of care.[55] For example, VA regulations do not allow VA pharmacies to fill prescriptions issued by non-VA prescribers except in limited circumstances.[56]

Prescriptions ordered by VA prescribers are filled through pharmacies located at VA facilities or through VA mail order pharmacies and are captured in the VA's integrated electronic health record. If veterans fill prescriptions outside the VA system, their VA providers may not be aware of these prescriptions, which could potentially affect treatment decisions. The same principle (i.e., all providers needing to know about all care received) applies to treatments other than prescriptions as well.

POLICY LEVERS AVAILABLE TO CONGRESS

Policy levers Congress might use to encourage adoption of specific strategies for increasing VAFQHC collaboration include (1) oversight, (2) an incentive fund, (3) directed spending, (4) statutory mandates, and (5) watchful waiting. Congress may also consider a combination of these levers should it wish to enhance VA-FQHC collaboration. All of the policy levers discussed here may be applicable to any number of other potential collaborations between VA and non-VA facilities.

The textbox provides examples of past congressional actions that have encouraged or facilitated VA-FQHC collaboration.[59] Each of the policy levers is then discussed briefly.

Examples of Past Congressional Actions to Encourage VA-FQHC Collaboration

- 106th Congress: The Departments of Veterans Affairs and Housing and Urban Development, and Independent Agencies, Appropriations Act, 2000 (P.L. 106-74; H.Rept. 106-379) report "urge[d] the VA to partner with existing, [FQHCs] to provide outpatient primary and preventive health care services to area veterans in their home communities" and stated that doing so "would greatly enhance access to quality health care for veterans living in remote areas."[57]
- 109th Congress: Section 212 of the Veterans Benefits, Health Care, and Information Technology Act of 2006 (P.L. 109-461) established the VA's Office of Rural Health (ORH) to coordinate efforts to improve health care for rural veterans.
- 111th Congress: The Consolidated Security, Disaster Assistance, and Continuing Appropriations Act, 2009 (P.L. 110-329) and the Consolidated Appropriations Act, 2010 (P.L. 111-117) appropriated $533 million to improve health care for rural veterans. According to the VA Inspector General, in FY2009, ORH received $250 million to implement new rural health outreach and delivery initiatives. In FY2010, ORH received an additional $250 million for rural health care, $30 million to open 51 rural Community Based Outpatient Clinics, and $3 million for rural hiring initiatives.[58]
- 111th Congress: The Caregivers and Veterans Omnibus Health Services Act of 2010 (P.L. 111-163) authorizes, among other things, demonstration projects on alternatives for expanding care for veterans in rural areas. The law also authorizes ORH to carry out demonstration projects that would establish partnerships between the VA and the Centers for Medicare and Medicaid Services to coordinate care for veterans in rural areas at critical access hospitals (i.e., small rural hospitals eligible to receive higher Medicare payments).

  This law also authorizes ORH to establish partnerships between the VA and HHS to coordinate care for veterans in rural areas at community health centers (i.e., FQHCs), and authorizes $5 million for FY2010 and subsequent fiscal years to conduct these demonstration projects.

- 112th Congress: The Consolidated Appropriations Act, 2012 (P.L. 112-74) includes $250 million to improve access and quality of care for veterans residing in rural areas.

Source: CRS analysis of legislation and U.S. Department of Veterans Affairs, Office of Inspector General, Veterans Health Administration Audit of the Office of Rural Health, Report No:10-02461-154, April 29, 2011.

Oversight

Congress has oversight of executive branch agencies, which it may leverage to encourage VAFQHC collaboration. For example, on the topic of access to mental health care services for veterans, Congress has conducted oversight hearings and requested reports from both GAO and the VA's Office of Inspector General.[60]

Congress may consider holding a hearing (or a series of hearings) on topics related to VA collaboration with FQHCs. Congress may also consider requesting a report evaluating the feasibility of increased collaboration between the VA and FQHCs, to be undertaken by the VA, GAO, or another entity. Such oversight might motivate the VA to address some of the considerations discussed in this report, even in the absence of other congressional activity.

Incentive Fund

Congress may consider appropriating funds to establish incentive funds to encourage or facilitate specified activities. For example, on the topic of collaboration between the VA and the Department of Defense (DOD), Congress used its authority to establish an incentive fund to increase VA-DOD collaboration.[61]

Congress may consider establishing an incentive fund to encourage the VA to contract with FQHCs. Such funds might be used, for example, to provide technical assistance to enable FQHCs to meet VA contracting requirements (e.g., to defray the cost of accreditation) or to enable the VA to manage the additional contracts.

Directed Spending

Congress may also consider using the appropriations process to direct funding for specific purposes. For example, on the topic of VA mental health care, the Consolidated Security, Disaster Assistance, and Continuing Appropriations Act, 2009 (P.L. 110-329) required the VA to spend at least $3.8 billion for mental health care.[62] Congress may consider employing a similar approach to direct that a certain amount of the VA's appropriation be spent on contracts with FQHCs. Such directed spending for the purpose of VA-FQHC collaboration might address VA funding considerations.

Statutory Mandates

Congress can mandate that executive agencies undertake certain activities. For example, Congress required the VA to coordinate with the Indian Health Service to provide care to American Indian and Alaska Native veterans who seek care at the Indian Health Service.[63] Congress may consider mandating that the VA engage in more collaboration with FQHCs. Congress may also consider requiring the VA to implement some or all of the recommendations in the NACHC report on VA-FQHC collaboration.[64]

Watchful Waiting

Watchful waiting is an option that is always available to Congress. If, for example, Congress determines that current levels of VA-FQHC collaboration are adequate, or that ongoing initiatives are sufficient to increase VA-FQHC collaboration to an adequate level, Congress may allow the current situation to unfold without further congressional involvement.

CONCLUSION

This report uses FQHCs as an extended example of existing facilities with which the VA might collaborate to provide services for veterans who do not live near a VA facility. This example forms the basis for discussing considerations that might come into play when the VA and non-VA providers (e.g., FQHCs) are deciding whether to collaborate, as well as for discussing policy levers available to Congress. Collaboration with non-VA providers is one option available to Congress should it want to expand access to rural veterans. Other available options include, but are not limited to, building new VA facilities (either CBOCs or VAMCs), expanding telehealth services,[65] expanding the VA's Fee Basis Care program,[66] or expanding VA travel benefits.[67]

APPENDIX A. EXISTING VA-FQHC COLLABORATIONS

A 2011 VA-commissioned report by the National Association of Community Health Centers (NACHC) recommended specific strategies to encourage VA-FQHC collaboration, several of which address considerations discussed in this CRS report (e.g., sufficiency of reimbursements).[68] Strategies such as those recommended in the NACHC report may be adopted without congressional action; however, Congress may choose to encourage, discourage, mandate, or prohibit specific strategies using a range of policy levers.

Some recommendations from the NACHC report are summarized in the *text box.*

Examples of Recommendations from VA-FQHC Collaborations Report

By request of the VA, the National Association of Community Health Centers and Atlas Research prepared a report entitled *Collaboration with Rural Community Health Centers VISN 5*. Although the report is specific to VISN 5 (the District of Columbia, Maryland, northern Virginia, and eastern West Virginia), the recommendations may be broadly applicable across the VA health care system. Below are some examples of relevant recommendations:

- Pilot test different payment mechanisms to reimburse FQHCs for services provided to veterans.
- Explore the feasibility of making VA electronic health records interoperable with FQHC record systems and develop quality indicators and other metrics to share data on veterans who access both VA facilities and FQHCs.
- Investigate models for coordination between the VA and FQHCs.

- Develop telehealth linkages between FQHCs and the VA for behavioral health care for veterans.
- Implement various strategies to increase FQHC provider education and awareness of the VA patient population.
- Consider contracting with FQHCs to act as CBOCs in areas where the VA population is too small to sustain a VA-operated facility.

Source: Adapted from National Association of Community Health Centers and Atlas Research, Collaboration with Rural Community Health Centers VISN 5, Task 4: Final Report, June 2011, pp. 66-67.

In addition to the 2011 commissioned report, the VA has also pursued contracts with FQHCs. See *Table A-1.*

Table A-1. Contracts Between the VA and Federally Qualified Health Centers (FQHCs)
Contracts for Counseling Services, by Veterans Integrated Service Network (VISN)

Veterans Integrated Service Network (VISN)[a]	Number of Current Contracts
VISN 1 New England Healthcare System	6
VISN 2: VA Health Care Upstate New York	5
VISN 3: VA NY/NJ Veterans Healthcare Network	1
VISN 4: VA Healthcare - VISN 4	2
VISN 6: VA Mid-Atlantic Health Care Network	1
VISN 7: VA Southeast Network	7
VISN 8: VA Sunshine Healthcare Network	1
VISN 17: VA Heart of Texas Health Care Network	5
VISN 18: VA Southwest Health Care Network	3
VISN 19: Rocky Mountain Network	8
VISN 20: Northwest Network	7
VISN 21: Sierra Pacific Network	4
VISN 22: Desert Pacific Healthcare Network	2
Total	52

Source: U.S. Department of Veterans Affairs, Veterans Health Administration. Information provided in response to a Congressional Research Service request.

[a] VISNs, geographically defined networks within the VA health care system, are described in Appendix B. VISNs not included in the table do not currently (as of February 2012) have contracts with FQHCs.

APPENDIX B. BACKGROUND ON HEALTH CARE DELIVERED OR FINANCED BY THE DEPARTMENT OF VETERANS AFFAIRS

The following appendix presents a brief overview of the VA health care system. This overview is not meant to be a comprehensive description; instead, it focuses on aspects of the VA health care system that are most relevant to collaboration with FQHCs.

Overview of VA Health Care

The VA operates the nation's largest integrated health care delivery system, with more than 258,000 full-time equivalent employees[69] providing care to more than 5.5 million patients.[70] The organization of the VA health system, the services available, and their costs, among other factors influence the VA's decisions to enter into contracts with outside providers and the need for such contracts. The following sections briefly summarize the VA health care system, including (1) enrollment, medical benefits, and cost-sharing; (2) budgetary and decision-making authority; (3) delivery of care; and (4) financing of care from non-VA providers.

VA Enrollment, Medical Benefits, and Cost-Sharing

The VA health care system is generally a provider—rather than a financer—of health care services; however, like public programs and private companies that finance health care (e.g., Medicare or private health insurance), the VA has enrollment criteria, a medical benefits package, and cost-sharing arrangements. VA enrollment, medical benefits, and cost-sharing have implications for the potential scope, feasibility, and cost of collaboration between the VA and non-VA providers such as FQHCs.

Formal collaborative arrangements between the VA and non-VA providers would apply only to veterans enrolled in VA health care. In general, eligibility for enrollment in VA health care operates through a system of eight priority groups, based on veteran status,[71] presence of service-connected disabilities[72] or exposures,[73] income,[74] and/or other factors, such as status as a former prisoner of war or receipt of a Purple Heart. Once enrolled in the VA health care system, a veteran remains enrolled and does not have to reapply, even if the veteran's priority group changes (due, for example, to a change in income).

Alignment between medical benefits available from the VA and services available from non-VA providers may affect the feasibility of collaboration. All enrolled veterans are offered a standard medical benefits package.[75] In addition to the standard medical benefits package, some veterans may receive additional benefits (e.g., dental care) based on their priority group or service-connected condition.

A veteran's out-of-pocket cost of care from a non-VA provider may vary depending on whether the care is provided under formal collaboration with the VA. Veterans do not pay premiums or enrollment fees to receive care from the VA; however, some veterans may incur out-of-pocket costs for VA care related to conditions that are not service-connected.[76] Whether enrolled in VA health care or not, veterans may have other sources of care (including, but not limited to, FQHCs), as well as various sources of health care financing (including, but not limited to, Medicare or private health insurance).[77] When a veteran receives health care services that are neither provided by the VA nor financed by the VA, the veteran or a third party payer would be responsible for the cost of the services.

VA Decision-Making Authority and Budgetary Responsibility

VA decision-making authority and budgetary responsibility are somewhat decentralized such that decisions about collaboration may be influenced by considerations at multiple levels within the agency. While policies and guidelines developed at VA headquarters are applied throughout the VA health care system, basic decision-making authority is delegated to 21 geographically defined Veterans Integrated Service Networks (VISNs).[78] (See *Figure B-1* for a map of the VISNs.) Within each VISN, some authority—which may include decision making on collaboration—is further delegated to facility directors.

Each year the VA allocates a majority of congressionally appropriated funds for health care services to the VISNs using a formula-based system called the Veterans Equitable Resource Allocation (VERA).[79] Each VISN's VERA allocation is based primarily on the number of patients treated; the complexity of each patient's treatment; adjustments for regional variations in labor and contract costs; and budgetary need for education support, research support, equipment, and non-recurring maintenance. The VERA allocation takes into account each VISN's unique characteristics and is adjusted to account for those veterans who receive care in more than one VISN. The VA provides each VISN director a standardized model that proposes allocations to facilities within the VISN; the VISN director has the flexibility to adjust the proposed allocations.[80] Facility directors bear responsibility for managing their facilities' budgets.

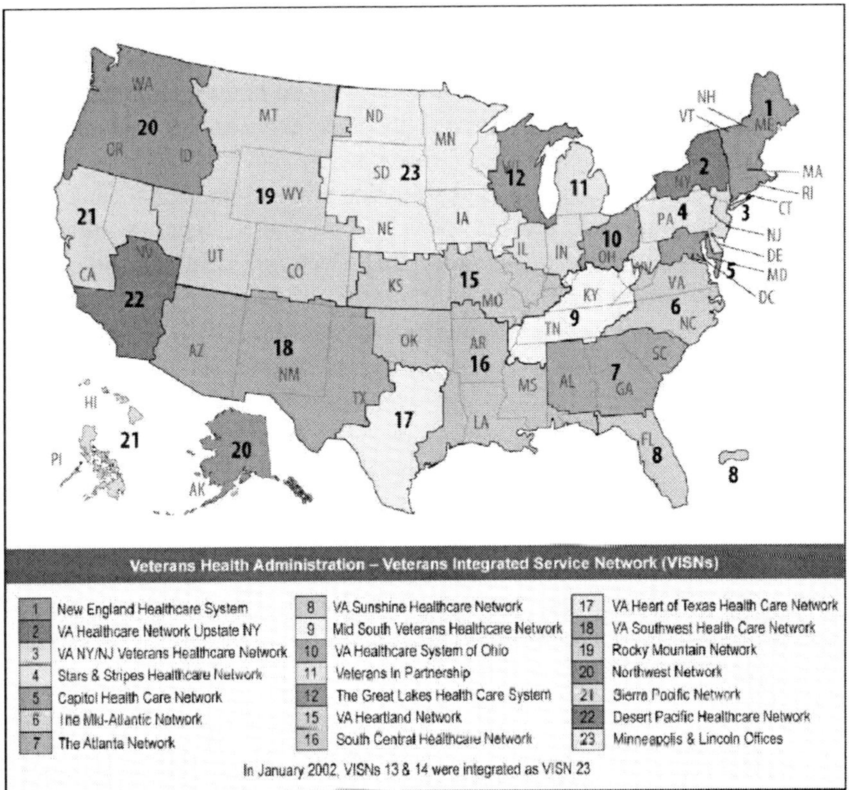

Source: U.S. Department of Veterans Affairs, adapted by the Congressional Research Service.

Figure B-1. Veterans Integrated Service Networks (VISNs).

VA Delivery of Care

The services available at VA facilities, their locations, and the extent to which they are integrated are important for understanding the system available to rural veterans and any gaps that might be filled through collaboration. The VA health care delivery system includes medical and nonmedical facilities, which differ in both the services available and the use of an integrated electronic health record. Each of these components of the VA health care delivery system is described briefly below.

VA medical facilities include more than 150 VA medical centers (VAMCs), 800 community-based outpatient clinics (CBOCs), and a range of other types of facilities (e.g., nursing homes). In general, VAMCs are located in urban areas and provide a wide range of primary and specialty care services, including both outpatient and inpatient (medical and surgical) care. CBOCs function as satellites of VAMCs, expanding the geographic reach of the VA health care system while generally offering a more limited range of services than VAMCs.[81] CBOCs are intended to make services available closer to where veterans reside, relative to VAMCs; nearly half of CBOCs are located in rural areas.[82] Generally all CBOCs provide primary care and mental health services; some may also provide specialty care and subspecialty care.[83] All VAMCs and CBOCs share an integrated electronic health record, which allows VA providers to view documentation of a patient's treatment regardless of which facility provided the treatment.

Alongside the VA's network of medical facilities, some 300 readjustment counseling centers (Vet Centers) provide psychosocial services—but not medical care. As of FY2012, the VA also has 70 Mobile Vet Centers, which were created in 2009 as part of a pilot program to improve access to services for veterans in rural areas.[84] Vet Centers, which have different eligibility criteria than the rest of the VA health care system, provide veterans and their families with services such as screening and counseling for PTSD or substance use disorders, bereavement counseling, military sexual trauma counseling, marital and family counseling, and employment and educational counseling. Vet Centers do not share the electronic health record used by VAMCs and CBOCs.

VA Financing of Care from Non-VA Providers

The VA is statutorily required to provide VA-enrolled veterans with access to timely and quality medical care;[85] meeting this requirement may involve the use of non-VA providers paid by the VA. Two mechanisms for VA financing of care from non-VA providers—contracted care and fee basis care—are described briefly below.[86] Contracted care is more likely than fee basis care to be used in formal VA-FQHC collaborations.

Contracted Care

The VA has statutory authority to contract for services from non-VA providers when essential medical services are not readily available within the VA's integrated health care system.[87] The VA may enter into contracts for the purchase of health care services with any health care provider (including an

FQHC).[88] The VA generally purchases health care services that may not be readily available at VAMCs; examples include radiation therapy, diagnostic radiology, cardiology, cardiovascular surgery, and orthopedics.[89]

A specific use of the VA's contracting authority is to enter into contracts with non-VA providers (including FQHCs) to establish contractor-operated CBOCs.[90] In general, contractor-operated CBOCs are open at least five days a week, for a minimum of 40 hours. The contractor is required to

- provide staff, facilities, equipment, supplies, and all administrative functions;
- meet both VA standards and The Joint Commission accreditation standards;[91] and
- use the VA's electronic health record to document all patient care.

The VA generally pays contractor-operated CBOCs a monthly fee for each enrolled patient; payments for each new enrollee begin during the month of the patient's first visit.[92]

Fee Basis Care

The VA may reimburse non-VA providers (including FQHCs) for health care services rendered to veterans on a fee-for-service basis (commonly referred to as Fee Basis Care); this program is only used under certain circumstances and does not represent a formal collaborative relationship between the VA and a particular non-VA provider (such as an FQHC). Specifically, Fee Basis Care is authorized under the following circumstances: (1) when a clinical service cannot be provided at a VAMC; (2) when a veteran is unable to access VA health care facilities due to geographic inaccessibility; or (3) in emergencies when delays could lead to life-threatening situations.[93] The VA's Fee Basis Care program is partially centralized (at the VISN level) and partially decentralized (at the VAMC level); in practice, most VAMCs independently administer the Fee Basis Care Program.[94]

Although fee basis care may include inpatient care, emergency care, medical transportation, and dental services, it is used predominantly to provide outpatient care.[95] The Fee Basis Care Program Office at the local VAMC pre-authorizes outpatient fee basis care if the care is determined to be appropriate, the veteran is eligible for the program, and an appropriate justification has been provided. Once outpatient fee basis care has been authorized, the veteran selects a provider and receives the service. The provider then sends a claim to the Fee Basis Care Program Office at the authorizing VAMC. After the claim is reviewed and processed, the non-VA provider receives payment electronically.[96]

APPENDIX C. BACKGROUND ON FEDERALLY QUALIFIED HEALTH CENTERS (FQHCS)

The following appendix presents a brief overview of the FQHCs. This overview is not meant to be a comprehensive description; instead, it focuses on aspects of the FQHCs that are most relevant to collaboration with the VA.

Any entity that receives a grant under the Federal Health Center Program[97] is called a health center; to be designated a federally qualified health center (FQHC), a health center must be (1) enrolled as a provider in the Medicare and Medicaid programs and (2) certified as an FQHC by the Centers for Medicare & Medicaid Services (CMS), making it eligible for generally higher Medicare and Medicaid payment rates.[98] The terms health center and FQHC are often used interchangeably, because most health centers receive the FQHC designation. The following sections describe the basic requirements to receive a Federal Health Center grant; these basic requirements affect, amongst other things, the services available and the location of facilities that, in turn, may affect collaboration with the VA.[99]

FQHCs are funded by grants authorized in Section 330 of the Public Health Service Act (PHSA), which establishes the requirements for entities to receive a grant; the alignment of these granting requirements and VA contracting requirements may affect collaboration. The grants awarded to support FQHCs are administered by the Health Resources and Services Administration (HRSA) within the Department of Health and Human Services (HHS). Health centers receiving a grant must, among other things: (1) offer specific health services; (2) provide services to all individuals in a given area regardless of their ability to pay, have an established fee schedule, and collect reimbursements for individuals enrolled in public or private insurance programs; and (3) be located in specific geographic areas.

Health Service Requirements

PHSA Section 330 requires that a health center provide certain services; the alignment of these required services with the VA basic medical benefits package may affect the feasibility of a VAFQHC collaboration. Specifically, FQHCs must provide primary, preventive, and emergency health services.[100] Primary health services are those provided by primary care physicians[101] or physician extenders (e.g., nurse practitioners) to diagnose, treat, or refer patients and include relevant diagnostic laboratory and radiology services. Preventive health services include well-child care, prenatal and postpartum care, immunization, family planning, health education, and preventive dental care. Emergency health services refer to the requirement that a health center have defined arrangements with outside providers for emergency cases that the center is not equipped to treat and for after-hours care.

In addition to these three types of services (primary, preventive, and emergency), a health center must meet a variety of other service requirements. A health center must provide diabetes self-management training for patients with diabetes or renal disease. Health center providers must also have admitting privileges at one or more hospitals located near the health center to ensure care continuity for hospitalized health center patients. A health center is required to provide enabling services, such as transportation for individuals residing in each center's service area who have difficulty accessing the center, translation services, and health education. A health center may also provide supplemental services such as additional dental care, mental health services, or substance abuse treatment. The supplemental services provided vary by health center, and this variation may affect collaboration with the VA or other entities.

Fee Schedule and Collection Requirements

FQHCs provide care to all individuals (including veterans) regardless of their ability to pay for services, and are required to collect reimbursements for the cost of these services; therefore all veterans have access to FQHCs, but payment for services received may be a consideration in VAFQHC collaboration. A health center must establish a fee schedule that takes into account local rates for health services and the costs that the health center incurs providing services. The health center is then required to establish a separate discounted fee schedule, which is then further discounted or waived based on a patient's ability to pay. Ability to pay is determined by the patient's income relative to the federal poverty level. The statute requires that individuals whose income is above 200% of the federal poverty level pay full charges, while individuals whose incomes are at or below 100% of the federal poverty level pay only nominal fees.[102]

A health center must seek reimbursement from third party payers such as private insurance plans, Medicare, Medicaid, and the State Children's Health Insurance Program (CHIP). The VA is not technically a third party payer (although it functions as such when reimbursing for fee basis care or contracting for services); therefore, FQHCs are not required to seek reimbursements from the VA. Instead, in absence of formal collaboration with the VA, an FQHC would seek reimbursement directly from the veteran (or a third-party payer if available) who receives care at the FQHC.

Location Requirements

PHSA Section 330 requires that a health center be located in a medically underserved area or serve a medically underserved population (see *text box*).[103] As a result of this requirement, many health centers are located in rural areas, which may make them candidates for collaboration with the VA to improve access for rural veterans.

Medically Underserved Areas/Populations

Medically Underserved Areas (MUA): Areas of varying size—whole counties, groups of contiguous counties, civil divisions, or a group of urban census tracts—where residents have a shortage of health care services.

Medically Underserved Populations (MUPs): Groups that face economic, cultural, or linguistic barriers to accessing health care.

Source: HRSA, Bureau of Primary Care, Shortage Designations, at http://bhpr.hrsa.gov/shortage/index.html.

Because the definition of a medically underserved area/population encompasses both urban and rural areas, FQHCs are located throughout the United States. The map (*Figure C-1*) below shows that FQHCs are dispersed throughout the country with each state having at least one FQHC. The requirements for FQHCs to be located in medically underserved areas may mean that they are located in rural areas where veterans reside.

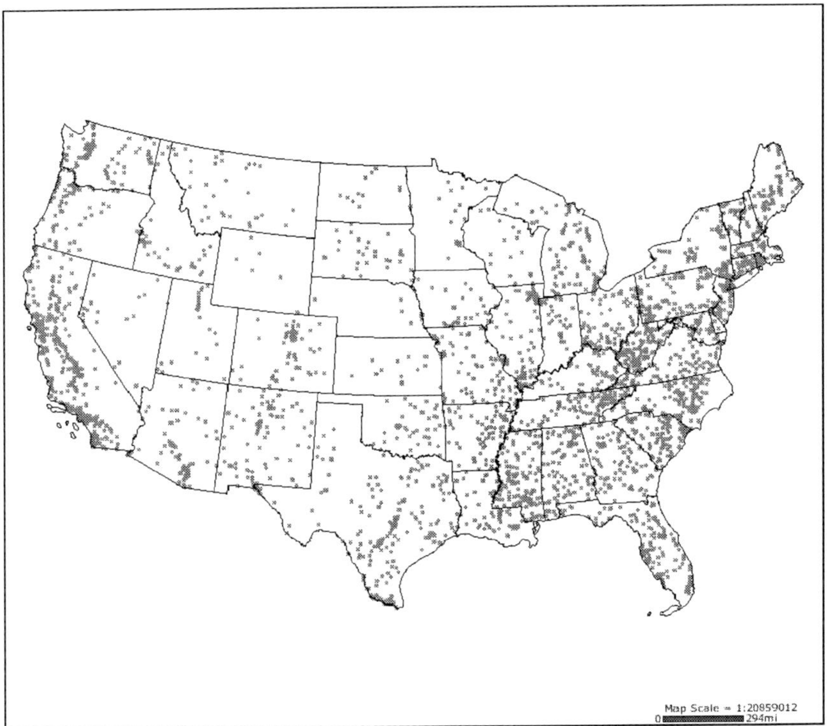

Source: Rural Assistance Center, at http://www.raconline.org/racmaps/#fqhc. Map is based on data obtained from the Center for Medicare & Medicaid Services, Quarter 2, 2011.

Note: This map does not depict Alaska or Hawaii, although both states have FQHCs.

Figure C-1. Federally Qualified Health Centers (FQHCs).

End Notes

[1] 38 U.S.C. §7301.

[2] U.S. Department of Veterans Affairs, *FY2013 Budget Submission, Medical Programs and Information Technology Programs,* Volume 2 of 4, February 2012, p. 1A-3.

[3] U.S. Department of Veterans Affairs (VA), Veterans Health Administration (VHA), Office of Rural Health (ORH), *Fact Sheet: Information about the Office of Rural Health and Rural Veterans*, April 2012, http://www.ruralhealth.va.gov/docs/ORH_General FactSheet_ April2012.pdf. The VA uses a three-tier classification system for population density: urban, rural, and highly rural. The system is based partly on the U.S. Census definitions of urban and rural; however, the VA divides the Census-designated rural areas into two categories, rural and highly rural (i.e., counties with fewer than 7 civilian residents per square mile). The VA designation of highly rural areas is similar to the designation that the Health

Resources and Services Administration (HRSA) uses when giving priority to "sparsely populated areas" in competition for Federally Qualified Health Center sites; see 42 U.S.C. §254b(p) and discussion in CRS Report R42433, *Federal Health Centers*, by Elayne J. Heisler.

[4] VA, VHA, ORH, *About Rural Veterans*, http://www.ruralhealth.va.gov/about/rural-veterans.asp. Many of the issues that rural veterans face are similar to the health care needs and access issues that all rural populations face. See, for example, United States Department of Agriculture, Economic Research Service, "Amber Waves June 2010— Findings—Rural Populations Have Higher Rates of Chronic Disease," press release, June 2010, http://www.ers.usda.gov/AmberWaves/June10/Findings/RuralPopulationsDisease.htm.

[5] VA, VHA, ORH, *About Rural Veterans*, http://www.ruralhealth.va.gov/about/rural-veterans.asp.

[6] The VA provides travel benefits to veterans; see CRS Report R41626, *Veterans Affairs Beneficiary Travel Program: Questions and Answers*, by Carol D. Davis.

[7] The VA has adapted the Institute of Medicine's (IOM's) definition of primary care, which defines primary care as "the provision of integrated, accessible health care services by clinicians who are accountable for addressing a large majority of personal health care needs, developing a sustained partnership with patients, and practicing in the context of family and community." See Department of Veterans Affairs, Veterans Health Administration, *Primary Care Standards*, VHA Directive 2012-011, April 11, 2012.

[8] Alan N. West et al., "Defining 'Rural' for Veterans' Health Care Planning," *The Journal of Rural Health*, no. 26 (2010), p. 301–309.

[9] Ibid.

[10] "Conference Report on H.R. 2684 Departments of Veterans Affairs and Housing and Urban Development, and Independent Agencies Appropriations Act, 2000," *Congressional Record*, October 13, 1999, p. H10005.

[11] Section 212 of the Veterans Benefits, Health Care, and Information Technology Act of 2006 (P.L. 109-461) established the VA's Office of Rural Health (ORH).

[12] The Caregivers and Veterans Omnibus Health Services Act of 2010 (P.L. 111-163) authorizes, among other things, several demonstration projects related to care for veterans in rural areas.

[13] This program was authorized in Section 403 of the Veterans' Mental Health and Other Care Improvements Act of 2008 (P.L. 110–387, enacted on October 10, 2008).

[14] See, for example, Consolidated Security, Disaster Assistance, and Continuing Appropriations Act, 2009 (P.L. 110- 329); Consolidated Appropriations Act, 2010 (P.L. 111-117), Consolidated Appropriations Act, 2012 (P.L. 112-74), and Consolidated and Further Continuing Appropriations Act, 2013 (P.L. 113-6).

[15] This is one of many options available. For example, under 38 U.S.C. §8111, the VA is authorized to enter into agreements to share health care resources with the Department of Defense (DOD); this provision may be used to establish Community Based Outpatient Clinics (CBOCs) at DOD facilities using personnel from DOD, VA, or both. Congress has also required the VA to coordinate with the Indian Health Service; see 25 U.S.C. §1645; see also description of Sec. 154 in CRS Report R41630, *The Indian Health Care Improvement Act Reauthorization and Extension as Enacted by the ACA: Detailed Summary and Timeline*, by Elayne J. Heisler; and U.S. Department of Veteran's Affairs, "VA and Indian Health Service Announce National Reimbursement Agreement," press release, December 6, 2012.

[16] National Association of Community Health Centers and Atlas Research, *Collaboration with Rural Community Health Centers VISN 5*, Task 4: Final Report, June 2011.

[17] Rural areas may also have "rural health clinics," which are outpatient facilities that provide primary care services to rural populations. Unlike FQHCs these facilities do not receive federal grants; instead they are designated as "rural health clinics" and made eligible for a higher Medicare payment rate. Although this designation gives the federal government some leverage over rural health clinics, they are not required to meet FQHC requirements, such as the requirement to provide specific services or to meet quality assurance standards. For more information on rural health clinics, see Center for Medicare & Medicaid Services, "Rural Health Clinic Fact Sheet," press release, June 2007, https://www.cms.gov/mln products/downloads/rhcfactsheet.pdf.

[18] CRS products on Benefits for Veterans, including the VA health care system, can be accessed at http://www.crs.gov/ pages/subissue.aspx?cliid=2179.

[19] 38 U.S.C. §7301.

[20] Overall, VA decision-making authority and budgetary responsibility are somewhat decentralized such that decisions about collaboration may be influenced by considerations at multiple levels within the agency. While policies and guidelines developed at VA headquarters are applied throughout the VA health care system, basic decision-making authority is delegated to 21 geographically defined Veterans Integrated Service Networks (VISNs). (See *Figure B-1* in *Appendix B* for a map of the VISNs.) Within each VISN, some authority—which may include decision making on collaboration—is further delegated to facility directors.

[21] An FQHC must seek reimbursement from third party payers such as private health insurers, Medicare, Medicaid, and the State Children's Health Insurance Program (CHIP). The VA is not considered a third party payer for this purpose; therefore, an FQHC is not required to seek reimbursements from the VA. Instead, an FQHC would seek reimbursement directly from the veteran (or a third party payer if available).

[22] 42 C.F R. 51c.303(f) and Section 330(k)(3)(G)(i) of the Public Health Service Act (PHSA).

[23] Fee basis care is described in greater depth in CRS Report R41065, *Veterans Health Care: Project HERO Implementation*, by Sidath Viranga Panangala.

[24] 38 U.S.C. §§1703, 1725, and 1728.

[25] The VA's Fee Basis Care program is partially centralized (at the Veterans Integrated Service Network (VISN) level and partially decentralized (at the VAMC level); in practice, most VAMCs independently administer the Fee Basis Care Program. See 38 U.S.C. §§1703, 1725, and 1728.

[26] 38 U.S.C. §§1703, 1725, and 1728.

[27] 38 U.S.C. §§8151-8153 delineates the VA's contracting authority. The VA may enter into contracts for the purchase of health care services with any health care provider (including an FQHC); see U.S. Department of Veterans Affairs, Office of Inspector General, *Evaluation of VHA Sole-Source Contracts with Medical Schools and Other Affiliated Institutions*, Report No. 05-01318-85, Washington, DC, February 16, 2005, p. 1.

[28] U.S. Department of Veterans Affairs, *Annual Report on Sharing of Health Care Resources Pursuant to the Provisions of 38 U.S.C. Section 8153, FY2008*, p. 3.

[29] The Veterans' Health Care Eligibility Reform Act (P.L. 104-262) authorized the VA to obtain health care resources by entering into contracts or other agreements with any health care facility, entity, or individual. For the VA's authority to enter into contracts to establish CBOCs, see 38 U.S.C. §8153, 38 U.S.C. §7409, and 38 U.S.C. §8111. Unless otherwise noted, information about contractor-operated CBOCs is from CRS Report R41044,

Veterans Health Administration: Community-Based Outpatient Clinics, by Sidath Viranga Panangala.

[30] The Joint Commission accredits and certifies health care organizations to ensure that certain standards are met. See http://www.jointcommission.org/about_us/about_the_joint_commission_main.aspx.

[31] Contractor-operated CBOCs are generally paid based on a Price Negotiation Memoranda, which describes the negotiated rate and the rationale for the procurement decision. A PNP is required by Department of Veterans Affairs, *Health Care Resources Contracting – Buying Title 38 U.S.C. 8153*, VA Directive 1663, August 10, 2006. Although generally a capitated rate is used, some contracts may pay the contractor-operated CBOC on a per visit basis. Specific payment rates are generally based on the Centers for Medicare & Medicaid Services (CMS) Medicare fee schedule.

[32] U.S. Department of Veterans Affairs, "Payment for Inpatient and Outpatient Health Care Professional Services at Non-Departmental Facilities and Other Medical Charges Associated With Non-VA Outpatient Care," 75 *Federal Register* 78901-78915, December 17, 2010.

[33] The Medicare FQHC payment rates are considered to be "higher" than the payment rates that physician practices receive, because they are cost-based and reflect a broader range of services than do payments to physician practices. See, for example, Department of Health Policy, School of Public Health and Health Services, The George Washington University, *Quality Incentives for Federally Qualified Health Centers, Rural Health Clinics and Free Clinics: A Report to Congress*, Washington, DC, January 23, 2012.

[34] U.S. Government Accountability Office, *Medicare Payments to Federally Qualified Health Centers*, GAO-10-576R, July 30, 2010; National Association of Community Health Centers, *A Sketch of Community Health Centers*, Chartbook, Washington, DC, 2009, http://www.nachc.com/client/documents/Chartbook%20FINAL%202009.pdf. The Patient Protection and Affordable Care Act (ACA, P.L. 111-148, as amended) required changes to the Medicare payment to FQHCs which, when implemented, may make Medicare reimbursements better reflect the cost of providing services. See Appendix B in CRS Report R42433, *Federal Health Centers*, by Elayne J. Heisler.

[35] 42 U.S.C. §254b.

[36] It is also possible that the patients who opt to receive services at FQHCs may have different health conditions than the patients who receive services at VA facilities. The VA allocation formula takes into account the complexity of each patient's treatment. Should this complexity differ between those receiving services within the VA and under contract and should this complexity not be reflected in VA records, it might affect the VA's allocation formula.

[37] Each year the VA allocates a majority of congressionally appropriated funds for health care services to the VISNs using a formula-based system called the Veterans Equitable Resource Allocation (VERA). Each VISN's VERA allocation is based primarily on the number of patients treated; the complexity of each patient's treatment; adjustments for regional variations in labor and contract costs; and budgetary need for education support, research support, equipment, and non-recurring maintenance. The VERA allocation takes into account each VISN's unique characteristics and is adjusted to account for those veterans who receive care in more than one VISN. A veteran receiving outpatient services must receive a medical history and physical examination at least once in a three-year period to remain as an active patient included in allocation calculations. For more information, see *Appendix B*.

[38] AMVETS, Disabled American Veterans, Paralyzed Veterans of America, and the Veterans of Foreign Wars, *Independent Budget, Fiscal Year 2013*, February 2012, p. 188. http://www.independentbudget.org/2013/IB_2013.pdf.

[39] Veterans' out-of-pocket costs may vary with factors such as income and service-connected disability.

[40] FQHCs are required to charge individuals without coverage based on a fee schedule that the FQHC develops and to collect reimbursements from individuals enrolled in private insurance plans or public coverage (e.g., Medicare or Medicaid). 42 U.S.C. §254b. Fees may be reduced or waived depending on patients' income, see http://bphc.hrsa.gov/ about/requirements/index.html.

[41] For example, FQHCs offer preventive dental services, but not all veterans are eligible for outpatient dental care through the VA. For detailed information on VA dental care, see http://www.va.gov/DENTAL/infoforpts.asp and http://www.va.gov/healthbenefits/assets/ documents/publications/ IB10-442.pdf#Dental. Section 510 of the Caregiver and Veterans Omnibus Health Services Act of 2010 (P.L. 111-163) required the VA to conduct a pilot program, by contract, for the purposes of offering a dental insurance plan to certain beneficiaries.

[42] Specifically, FQHCs must be located in Medically Underserved Areas (MUA): Areas of varying size—whole counties, groups of contiguous counties, civil divisions, or a group of urban census tracts—where residents have a shortage of health care services, or must serve Medically Underserved Populations (MUPs): Groups that face economic, cultural, or linguistic barriers to accessing health care. See Health Resources and Services Administration, Bureau of Primary Care, Shortage Designations, at http://bhpr.hrsa.gov/ shortage/index.html.

[43] Given that many FQHC patients are uninsured, some may seek care in emergency rooms because emergency rooms are required to provide care regardless of insurance status. Emergency room care is more expensive than care provided at an FQHC and may be less appropriate. For information on health outcomes and cost savings associated with FQHCs, see U.S. Government Accountability Office, *Hospital Emergency Departments: Health Center Strategies that May Help Reduce Their Use*, GAO-11-414R, April 11, 2011.

[44] CRS Report R42029, *Physician Supply and the Affordable Care Act*, by Elayne J. Heisler, 45 Roger A. Rosenblatt et al., "Shortages of Medical Personnel at Community Health Centers: Implications for Planned Expansion," *Journal of the American Medical Association*, vol. 295, no. 9 (March 2006), pp. 1042-1049; and U.S. Government Accountability Office, *Primary Care Professionals: Recent Supply Trends, Projections, and Valuation of Services*, GAO-08-472T, February 12, 2008.

[46] National Association of Community Health Centers, *The Struggle to Build a Strong Workforce at Health Centers*, Fact Sheet #0609, Washington, DC, 2009.

[47] Roger A. Rosenblatt et al., "Shortages of Medical Personnel at Community Health Centers: Implications for Planned Expansion," *Journal of the American Medical Association*, vol. 295, no. 9 (March 2006), pp. 1042-1049.

[48] The standard medical benefits package is described in detail in 38 C.F.R. §17.38. In addition to the standard medical benefits package, some veterans may receive additional benefits (e.g., dental care) based on their priority group or service-connected condition.

[49] 42 CFR 51c.102(h).

[50] 38 U.S.C. §7311.

[51] U.S. Department of Veterans Affairs, Veterans Health Administration, *Planning and Activating Community-Based Outpatient Clinics*, VHA Handbook 1006.1, May 19, 2004, p. 8.

[52] CRS Report R42433, *Federal Health Centers*, by Elayne J. Heisler.

[53] Recent work by GAO found that system compatibility was an issue in VA-DOD collaboration. See U.S. Government Accountability Office, *Department-Level Actions Needed to Assess Collaboration Performance, Address Barriers, and Identify Opportunities*, 12-992, September 28, 2012, http://www.gao.gov/products/GAO-12-992.

[54] 42 U.S.C. §254b.

[55] FQHCs may also receive increased Medicaid payments for using electronic health records. FQHCs are required to have their own record system, so an FQHC that contracts with the VA may have to ensure that its electronic health record system can be used under the contract and for the Medicaid incentive program; otherwise the FQHC would have to forgo the Medicaid incentive payments. For more information on Medicaid incentive payments for electronic health records see CRS Report R40161, *The Health Information Technology for Economic and Clinical Health (HITECH) Act*, by C. Stephen Redhead.

[56] For exceptions, see 38 CFR §17.96.

[57] "Conference Report on H.R. 2684 Departments of Veterans Affairs and Housing and Urban Development, and Independent Agencies Appropriations Act, 2000," *Congressional Record*, October 13, 1999, p. H10005.

[58] U.S. Department of Veterans Affairs, Office of Inspector General, *Veterans Health Administration Audit of the Office of Rural Health*, Report No:10-02461-154, Washington, DC, April 29, 2011, p. 1.

[59] The Executive Branch may also encourage or facilitate collaboration. For example, a 2012 Executive Order required that the VA and the Department of Defense to, among other things, use pilot projects to collaborate with community providers (including FQHCs) to provide timely mental health services to veterans, members of the armed forces, and their families. See Executive Order 13625, "Improving Access to Mental Health Services for Veterans, Service Members, and Military Families," 77 *Federal Register* 54783-54786, August 31, 2012.

[60] See, for example, U.S. Congress, Senate Committee on Veterans' Affairs, *VA Mental Health Care: Addressing Wait Times and Access to Care*, 112th Cong., 1st sess., November 30, 2011; U.S. Government Accountability Office, *VA Mental Health: Number of Veterans Receiving Care, Barriers Faced, and Efforts to Increase Access*, GAO-12-12, October 14, 2011, http://www.gao.gov/products/GAO-12-12; and U.S. Department of Veterans Affairs, Office of Inspector General, *Review of Veterans' Access to Mental Health Care*, Report Number 12-00900-168, April 23, 2012, http://www.va.gov/oig/publications/report-summary.asp?id=2654.

[61] See the Bob Stump National Defense Authorization Act of 2003 (P.L. 107-314); 38 U.S.C. §8111(d). The purpose of this fund is to provide seed money for innovative sharing initiatives with the goal of improving access to, and the cost-effectiveness of, the health care provided to veterans and active duty servicemembers. The DOD and the VA contribute $15 million each fiscal year (through FY2015) to the Fund from funds appropriated to the two departments. For a discussion of this collaboration, see U.S. Government Accountability Office, *Department-Level Actions Needed to Assess Collaboration Performance, Address Barriers, and Identify Opportunities*, 12-992, September 28, 2012, http://www.gao.gov/products/GAO-12-992.

62 See the CRS Report RL34598, *Veterans Medical Care: FY2009 Appropriations*, by Sidath Viranga Panangala.

63 See 25 U.S.C. §1645 described in Sec. 154 of CRS Report R41630, *The Indian Health Care Improvement Act Reauthorization and Extension as Enacted by the ACA: Detailed Summary and Timeline*, by Elayne J. Heisler. See also U.S. Department of Veteran's Affairs, "VA and Indian Health Service Announce National Reimbursement Agreement," press release, December 6, 2012.

64 National Association of Community Health Centers and Atlas Research, *Collaboration with Rural Community Health Centers VISN 5, Task 4: Final Report,* June 2011, pp. 66-67

65 This strategy is currently being used in collaborations between the VA and HHS; see Department of Health and Human Services, "Veterans in Rural Areas to Get Expanded Access to Health Care," press release, September 12, 2012, http://www.hhs.gov/news/press/2012pres/09/20120912b.html.

66 In late 2012, the VA initiated an effort to create a system-wide health care contracting strategy known as the Patient-Centered Community Care (PC3) initiative. It will provide eligible veterans coordinated access to care through a comprehensive network of non-VA providers who meet VA quality standards when the VA cannot provide care within its own facilities. The VA is scheduled to award PC3 contracts in April 2013. Briefing to Congressional Staff, Department of Veterans Affairs, Office of Congressional and Legislative Affairs, "Veterans Health Administration: Patient-Centered Community Care-PC3" March 8, 2013.

67 CRS Report R41626, *Veterans Affairs Beneficiary Travel Program: Questions and Answers*, by Carol D. Davis.

68 National Association of Community Health Centers and Atlas Research, *Collaboration with Rural Community Health Centers VISN 5, Task 4: Final Report,* June 2011, pp. 66-67.

69 U.S. Department of Veterans Affairs, *FY 2011 Performance and Accountability Report*, Washington, DC, November 15, 2011, p.I-31.

70 U.S. Department of Veterans Affairs, *FY2013 Budget Submission, Medical Programs and Information Technology Programs,* Volume 2 of 4, February 2012, p. 1A-3.

71 Veteran status is established by active-duty status in the U.S. Armed Forces and an honorable discharge or release from active military service. Generally, persons enlisting in one of the armed forces after September 7, 1980, and officers commissioned after October 16, 1981, must have completed two years of active duty or the full period of their initial service obligation to be eligible for VA health care benefits. Servicemembers discharged at any time because of service-connected disabilities are not held to this requirement. Veterans returning from combat operations are eligible to enroll for five years from the date of discharge without having to satisfy a means test or demonstrate a service-connected disability.

72 A service-connected disability is a disability that was incurred or aggravated in the line of duty in the U.S. Armed Forces (38 U.S.C. §101 (16)). The VA determines whether veterans have service-connected disabilities and, for those with such disabilities, assigns ratings from 0% to 100% based on the severity of the disability (38 C.F.R. §§4.1-4.31).

73 For example, veterans who may have been exposed to Agent Orange during the Vietnam War or veterans who may have diseases potentially related to service in the Gulf War may be eligible to receive care.

74 Veterans meeting certain income criteria may be eligible to enroll in the VA without a service-connected condition.

75 The standard medical benefits package is described in detail in 38 C.F.R. §17.38.

[76] 38 U.S.C. §1729. Veterans rated 50% or more service-connected disabled are exempt from all copayments.

[77] The VA is required to collect reasonable charges for medical care or services (including prescription drugs) from a third-party insurer if the care provided would be covered under a private insurance plan; however, the VA generally does not collect reimbursements from Medicare or Medicaid. 38 U.S.C. §1729(a)(2)(D); 38 C.F.R. §17.101(a)(1)(i) (2011). Some veterans may also be eligible to receive services either directly from the military health system or paid for by TRICARE, which purchases care for active duty servicemembers and other eligible beneficiaries (such as military retirees). For more information see CRS Report RL33537, *Military Medical Care: Questions and Answers*, by Don J. Jansen and Katherine Blakeley.

[78] Kenneth Kizer, John Demakis, and John Feussner, "Reinventing VA Health Care: Systematizing Quality Improvement and Quality Innovation." *Medical Care,* vol. 38, no. 6 (June 2000), Suppl 1:I7-16.

[79] For more information on appropriations for VA health care, see CRS Report R42518, *Veterans' Medical Care: FY2013 Appropriations*, by Sidath Viranga Panangala.

[80] U.S. Government Accountability Office, *VA Health Care: Need for More Transparency in New Resource Allocation Process and for Written Policies on Monitoring Resources*, GAO-11-426, April 29, 2011, p. 13.

[81] The VA also operates 6 independent outpatient clinics (which are not satellites of VAMCs and are not part of the VISN structure) and 10 mobile outpatient clinics. U.S. Department of Veterans Affairs, FY2013 Budget Submission, Medical Programs and Information Technology Programs, Volume 2 of 4, Feb. 2012, p. 1E-5.

[82] U.S. Department of Veterans Affairs, *Reaching Out to Three Million "Rural" Veterans*, August 16, 2012, http://www.va.gov/health/NewsFeatures/20120816a.asp.

[83] See CRS Report R41044, *Veterans Health Administration: Community-Based Outpatient Clinics*, by Sidath Viranga Panangala.

[84] U.S. Department of Veterans Affairs, *Vet Center: Services*, 2010, http://www.vetcenter.va.gov/Vet_Center_Services.asp; and U.S. Department of Veterans Affairs, "VA Deploying 20 New Mobile Vet Centers," press release, January 4, 2012, http://www1.va.gov/opa/pressrel/pressrelease.cfm?id=2241.

[85] 38 U.S.C. §7301.

[86] Fee basis care is described in greater depth in CRS Report R41065, *Veterans Health Care: Project HERO Implementation*, by Sidath Viranga Panangala.

[87] 38 U.S.C. §§8151-8153 delineates the VA's contracting authority.

[88] U.S. Department of Veterans Affairs, Office of Inspector General, *Evaluation of VHA Sole-Source Contracts With Medical Schools And Other Affiliated Institutions*, Report No. 05-01318-85, Washington, DC, February 16, 2005, p. 1.

[89] U.S. Department of Veterans Affairs, *Annual Report on Sharing of Health Care Resources Pursuant to the Provisions of 38 U.S.C. Section 8153, FY2008*, p. 3.

[90] The Veterans' Health Care Eligibility Reform Act (P.L. 104-262) authorized the VA to obtain health care resources by entering into contracts or other agreements with any health care facility, entity, or individual. For the VA's authority to enter into contracts to establish CBOCs, see 38 U.S.C. §8153, 38 U.S.C. §7409, and 38 U.S.C. §8111. Unless otherwise noted, information about contractor-operated CBOCs is from CRS Report R41044, *Veterans Health Administration: Community-Based Outpatient Clinics*, by Sidath Viranga Panangala.

[91] The Joint Commission accredits and certifies health care organizations to ensure that certain standards are met. See http://www.jointcommission.org/about_us/about_the_ joint_ commission_main.aspx.

[92] Although generally a capitated rate is used, some contracts may pay the contractor-operated CBOC on a per visit basis. Specific payment rates are generally based on the Centers for Medicare & Medicaid Services (CMS) Medicare fee schedule. A Price Negotiation Memorandum, which describes the negotiated rate and the rationale for the procurement decision, is required by Department of Veterans Affairs, *Health Care Resources Contracting – Buying: Title 38 U.S.C. 8153*, VA Directive 1663, August 10, 2006.

[93] 38 U.S.C. §§1703, 1725, and 1728. A recently released proposed rule that would extend this program and permit the VA to reimburse care that is provided to complete treatment for an episode of care that was provided by a non-VA providers. Previously, non-VA care was only authorized for necessary services required to complete treatment related to a VA-provided hospitalization. The new rule would permit reimbursement of services provided for up to 12 months after an episode of care and would permit this time period to be extended as needed. Department of Veterans Affairs, "Authorization of Non-VA Medical Services," 77 *Federal Register* 70967-70968, November 28, 2012.

[94] U.S. Department of Veterans Affairs, Office of Inspector General, *Audit of Veterans Health Administration's Non-VA Outpatient Fee Care Program*, Report No. 08-02901-185, Washington, DC, August 23, 2009.

[95] Ibid.

[96] Ibid.

[97] The Federal Health Center Program is authorized in Section 330 of the Public Health Service Act; 42 U.S.C. §254b.

[98] See discussion in Appendix B of CRS Report R42433, *Federal Health Centers*, by Elayne J. Heisler.

[99] For more information see CRS Report R42433, *Federal Health Centers*, by Elayne J. Heisler.

[100] 42 CFR 51c.102(h).

[101] The regulation defines primary care physicians as those in family practice, internal medicine, pediatrics, or obstetrics and gynecology.

[102] 42 C.F. R. 51c.303(f) and Section 330(k)(3)(G)(i) of the Public Health Service Act (PHSA).

[103] Section 5602 of the Patient Protection and Affordable Care Act (ACA, P.L. 111-148) required the Secretary of HHS to revise the criteria and methodology used to designate health professional shortage areas (HPSAs) and MUPs. The ACA also required that HHS appoint a committee to undertake this revision and publish a final rule with the new criteria. The committee released a report on October 1, 2011, see http://www.hrsa.gov/advisory committees/shortage/ nrmcfinalreport.pdf, but failed to reach a consensus; therefore, HRSA has discretion in using the committee's recommendation when undertaking rulemaking to revise the criteria and methodology used to designate HPSAs and MUPs. HRSA has not begun rulemaking in this area as of the date of this report's publication.

In: Veterans
Editor: Timothy C. Roberts

ISBN: 978-1-63117-046-1

Chapter 2

VA AND IHS: FURTHER ACTION NEEDED TO COLLABORATE ON PROVIDING HEALTH CARE TO NATIVE AMERICAN VETERANS*

United States Government Accountability Office

WHY GAO DID THIS STUDY

Native Americans who have served in the military may be eligible for health care services from both VA and IHS. To enhance health care access and the quality of care provided to Native American veterans, in 2010, these two agencies renewed and revised an MOU designed to improve their coordination and resource sharing related to serving these veterans. GAO was asked to examine how the agencies have implemented the MOU.

This report examines: (1) the extent to which the agencies have established mechanisms through which the MOU can be implemented and monitored; and (2) key challenges the agencies face in implementing the MOU and the progress made in overcoming them. To conduct this work, GAO interviewed VA and IHS officials and reviewed agency documents and reports. GAO also obtained perspectives of tribal communities through attendance at two tribal conferences; interviews with tribal leaders and other

* This is an edited, reformatted and augmented version of the Highlights of GAO-13-354, a report to congressional requesters, dated April, 2013.

tribal members, including veterans; and interviews with other stakeholders, such as health policy experts and consultants.

WHAT GAO RECOMMENDS

GAO recommends that the agencies take steps to improve the performance metrics used to assess MOU implementation and to develop better processes to consult with tribes. VA and the Department of Health and Human Services agreed with these recommendations.

WHAT GAO FOUND

The Department of Veterans Affairs (VA) and the Indian Health Service (IHS) have developed mechanisms to implement and monitor their memorandum of understanding (MOU); however, the performance metrics developed to assess its implementation do not adequately measure progress made toward its goals. VA and IHS have defined common goals for implementing the MOU and developed strategies to achieve them. They have also created two mechanisms to implement the MOU—12 workgroups with members from both agencies to address the goals of the MOU, and a Joint Implementation Task Force, comprised of VA and IHS officials, to oversee the MOU's implementation. These steps are consistent with practices that GAO has found enhance and sustain agency collaboration. The agencies have also developed three metrics aimed at measuring progress toward the MOU's goals. However, two of the three metrics are inadequate because their connection to any specific MOU goal is not clear and, while they include quantitative measures that tally the number of programs and activities increased or enhanced as a result of the MOU, they lack qualitative measures that would allow the agencies to assess the degree to which the desired results are achieved. The weaknesses in these metrics could limit the ability of VA and IHS managers to gauge progress and make decisions about whether to expand or modify their programs and activities.

VA and IHS face unique challenges associated with consulting with a large number of diverse, sovereign tribes to implement the MOU, and lack fully effective processes to overcome these complexities. VA and IHS officials told us the large number (566 federally recognized tribes) and differing customs and policy-making structures present logistical challenges in widespread implementation of the MOU within tribal communities. They also told us that tribal sovereignty—tribes' inherent right to govern and protect the health, safety, and welfare of tribal members—adds further complexity because tribes may choose whether or not to participate in MOU-related activities. Consistent with internal controls, VA and IHS have processes in place to consult with tribes on MOU- related activities through written correspondence and in-person meetings. However, according to tribal stakeholders GAO spoke with, these processes are often ineffective and have not always met the needs of the tribes, and the agencies have acknowledged that effective consultation has been challenging. For example, one tribal community expressed concern that agency correspondence is not always timely because it is sent to tribal leaders who are sometimes not the tribal members designated to take action on health care matters. Similarly, some tribal stakeholders told GAO that the agencies have not been responsive to tribal input and that sometimes they simply inform tribes of steps they have taken without consulting them. VA and IHS have taken steps to improve consultation with tribes. For example, VA has established an Office of Tribal Government Relations, through which it is developing relationships with tribal leaders and other tribal stakeholders. Additionally, in Alaska, VA has been consulting with a tribal health organization for insight on reaching tribes. However, given the concerns raised by the tribal stakeholders GAO spoke with, further efforts may be needed to enhance tribal consultation to implement and achieve the goals of the MOU.

ABBREVIATIONS

CMOP	Consolidated Mail Outpatient Pharmacy
EHR	electronic health record
HBPC	home-based primary care
IHS	Indian Health Service
MOU	memorandum of understanding
NCAI	National Congress of American Indians
OTGR	Office of Tribal Government Relations
VA	Department of Veterans Affairs

April 26, 2013

Congressional Requesters:

Native Americans (American Indians and Alaska Natives) have historically served in the military at a higher rate than any other ethnic group, according to the Department of Defense. Once separated from the military, some Native American veterans are eligible to receive health care services from both the Department of Veterans Affairs (VA) and the Indian Health Service (IHS), an agency within the Department of Health and Human Services.[1]

To improve the health status of Native American veterans through coordination, collaboration, and sharing of resources among VA, IHS, and tribes, in 2010, VA and IHS expanded upon a 2003 memorandum of understanding (MOU). This 2010 MOU outlined mutual goals for the agencies' collaboration and coordination of resources and care in providing health care services to Native American veterans. For example, it included provisions for joint contracts and purchasing agreements, sharing staff, ensuring providers in VA and IHS could access the electronic health records of shared patients, and the development of payment and reimbursement policies and mechanisms to support care delivered to Native American veterans eligible for care in both systems.

In a May 2012 congressional hearing, both VA and IHS reported that they have taken steps to collaborate to improve access to and quality of health care services for Native American veterans.[2] However, questions have been raised by members of Congress about the extent of collaboration between the two agencies. For example, a 2012 Senate report noted that stronger partnerships among VA, IHS, and tribally operated health facilities are essential to ensuring Native American veterans have access to health care services.[3] We were asked to examine how the agencies have implemented the MOU. In this report, we address the (1) extent to which VA and IHS have established mechanisms through which the MOU can be effectively implemented and monitored; and (2) key challenges that VA and IHS face in implementing the MOU, and the progress they have made in overcoming them.

To address both of these objectives, we reviewed the MOU and documentation related to the MOU's implementation, including periodic updates and descriptions of sharing agreements. We also reviewed the signed reimbursement agreement between VA and IHS as well as signed reimbursement agreements between VA and tribes.[4] We interviewed VA and

IHS officials, including VA's Director of the Office of Rural Health and Office of Tribal Government Relations, the IHS Chief Medical Officer, and leaders of 8 of 12 VA/IHS workgroups tasked with addressing and implementing the MOU to learn about the steps that have been taken to implement and monitor the MOU and any related challenges. We selected these eight workgroups because they were involved in addressing issues regarding agency coordination and sharing resources.[5]

To assess the MOU's implementation and related challenges, we took several actions to obtain the views of tribal communities. We attended a VA tribal consultation on MOU implementation at the National Indian Health Board Consumer Conference in Denver, Colorado, in September 2012, and attended the National Congress of American Indians (NCAI) Annual Conference in Sacramento, California, in October 2012. At the NCAI conference, we conducted listening sessions for tribal members to solicit their views on MOU implementation. We also interviewed various other tribal health representatives outside of the listening sessions and the conferences. In all, we interviewed 34 tribal members and other representatives (collectively referred to in this report as tribal stakeholders), including tribal leaders, tribal veterans, tribal health directors and administrators, and tribal health policy experts and consultants. The tribes represented in our interviews were geographically varied, including representation from 9 IHS Areas and 10 Veterans Integrated Service Networks and included representation from tribes that varied in size from approximately 500 members to 310,000 members. We cannot generalize findings from these interviews as representative of all tribal communities; however, we believe that patterns or issues identified in these interviews may illustrate issues that other tribes face as well.

To evaluate the extent to which VA and IHS have established mechanisms through which the MOU can be effectively implemented and monitored, we assessed this evidence against relevant criteria from our past work on interagency collaboration, practices from leading results-oriented public-sector organizations, and agency strategic planning.[6] To evaluate key challenges that VA and IHS face in implementing the MOU, and the progress they have made in overcoming them, we assessed this evidence against internal controls.[7]

We conducted this performance audit from July 2012 to April 2013 in accordance with generally accepted government auditing standards. Those standards require that we plan and perform the audit to obtain sufficient, appropriate evidence to provide a reasonable basis for our findings and conclusions based on our audit objectives. We believe that the evidence obtained provides a reasonable basis for our findings and conclusions based on our audit objectives.

BACKGROUND

Native American Veteran Demographics

While Native American veterans are geographically dispersed throughout the United States, the West and South regions contain the majority of the Native American veteran population, according to Census data. Some Native American veterans are members of the 566 federally recognized tribes that are distinct, independent political communities that possess certain powers of self-government, which we refer to as tribal sovereignty. Specifically, federally recognized tribes have government-to-government relationships with the United States, and are eligible for certain funding and services provided by the United States. In addition, some Native American veterans are members of the more than 400 Indian groups that are not recognized by the federal government (which we refer to in this report as non–federally recognized tribes).[8] Many—but not all—Native American veterans are dually eligible for health care services in VA and IHS. For example, a veteran who is a member of a non–federally recognized tribe may be eligible for VA health care services, but would not be eligible for IHS health care services.[9]

VA and IHS Structure and Benefits

VA is charged with providing health care services to the nation's veterans, and estimates that it will serve 6.3 million patients in fiscal year 2013. VA's fiscal year 2012 budget for medical care was approximately $54 billion. The department provides health care services at VA-operated facilities and through agreements with non-VA providers.[10] Veterans who served in the active military, naval or air service and who were discharged or released under conditions other than dishonorable are generally eligible for VA health care.

IHS is charged with providing health care to the approximately 2.1 million eligible Native Americans. IHS's fiscal year 2012 budget for medical care was approximately $3.9 billion. Similarly to VA, IHS provides health care services at IHS-operated facilities through direct care and pays for services from external providers through contract health services. In addition to IHS-operated facilities, some federally recognized tribes choose to operate their own health care facilities, which receive funding from IHS.[11] Like their IHS-operated counterparts, tribally operated facilities provide direct care services and pay for contract health services. IHS also provides funding through grants and contracts to nonprofit urban Native American organizations through the Urban Indian Health program in order to provide health care services to Native Americans living in urban areas.

VA and IHS Collaboration through Memorandums of Understanding

In 2003, VA and IHS signed an MOU to facilitate collaborative efforts in serving Native American veterans eligible for health care in both systems. In 2010, the agencies developed a more detailed MOU to further these efforts. The 2010 MOU contains provisions related to several areas of collaboration, including actions related to the following:

- *Joint contracts and purchasing agreements*: Development of standard, preapproved language for inclusion of one agency into contracts and purchasing agreements developed by the other agency; and processes to share information about sharing opportunities in early planning stages.
- *Sharing staff*: Establishment of joint credentialing and privileging, sharing specialty services, and arranging for temporary assignment of IHS Public Health Service commissioned officers to VA.
- *Electronic Health Record (EHR) access*: Establishment of standard mechanisms for VA providers to access records in IHS and tribally operated facilities, and vice versa, for patients receiving care in both systems.
- *Reimbursement*: Development of payment and reimbursement policies and mechanisms to support care delivered to dually eligible Native American veterans.

VA and IHS Tribal Consultation Policies

Executive Order 13175, issued on November 6, 2000, required federal agencies to establish regular and meaningful consultation and collaboration with Indian tribe officials in the development of federal policies that have tribal implications.[12] IHS issued a tribal consultation policy in 2006 to formalize the requirement to seek consultation and participation by Indian tribes in policy development and program activities. According to the policy, IHS will consult with Indian tribes to the extent practicable and permitted by law before any action is taken that will significantly affect Indian tribes. In November 2009, a Presidential Memorandum directed federal agencies to develop plans, after consultation with Indian tribes and tribal officials, for implementing the policies and directives of Executive Order 13175.[13] VA's plan included development of a tribal consultation policy, which the agency released in February 2011. VA's tribal consultation policy asserts that VA will establish meaningful consultation to develop, improve, or maintain partnerships with tribal communities. The policy states that consultation should be conducted before actions are taken but acknowledges there may not always be "sufficient time or resources to fully consult" on an issue.[14]

Best Practices and Internal Control Standards for Interagency Collaboration and Performance Monitoring

In past work we have reported on key practices to enhance and sustain interagency collaboration[15] including

- agreeing on roles and responsibilities;
- establishing compatible policies, procedures, and other means to operate across agency boundaries; and
- developing mechanisms to monitor, evaluate, and report on results.

Additionally, our past work has identified a range of mechanisms that the federal government uses to lead and implement interagency collaboration.[16] We found that regardless of the mechanisms used, there are key actions the government can take, including (1) having clear goals; (2) ensuring relevant participants are included in collaboration; and (3) specifying the resources—human, information, technology, physical, and financial—needed to initiate or sustain the collaboration. We have also found in past work on leading public-sector organizations and agency strategic planning that it is important to (1) define clear missions and desired outcomes; (2) use performance measures that are tangible, measurable, and clearly related to goals to gauge progress; and (3) use performance information as a basis for decision making.[17] Finally, internal control standards emphasize the importance of effective external communications that occur with groups that can have a serious effect on programs, projects, operations, and other activities, including budgeting and financing.[18]

VA and IHS Have Developed Mechanisms to Implement and Monitor the MOU, but Metrics to Monitor Performance Do Not Adequately Measure Progress toward MOU Goals

VA and IHS have documented common goals in their MOU, created 12 workgroups that are tasked with developing strategies to address the goals of the MOU, and created a Joint Implementation Task Force to coordinate tasks, develop implementation policy, and develop performance metrics and timelines—actions that are consistent with those we have found enhance and sustain agency collaboration. However, most of the performance metrics developed by VA and IHS to monitor the implementation of the MOU need to be more clearly related to the goals of the MOU in order to allow the agencies to gauge progress toward MOU goals.

VA and IHS Have Defined Common Goals and Created Mechanisms to Implement the MOU

Consistent with our past work on practices that can enhance and sustain collaboration, VA and IHS have defined common goals for implementing the MOU and developed specific strategies the agencies plan to take to achieve them. Table 1 summarizes the five goals in the 2010 MOU and selected strategies for implementing them.

VA and IHS have created two mechanisms to implement the MOU—workgroups and a Joint Implementation Task Force. We have reported that MOUs are most effective when they are regularly updated and monitored, actions that can be achieved by workgroups and task forces.[19]

Table 1. Goals and Associated Strategies in the Department of Veterans Affairs (VA) / Indian Health Service (IHS) 2010 Memorandum of Understanding (MOU)

MOU goal	Selected strategies to achieve goal
1. Increase access to and improve quality of health care and services to the mutual benefit of both agencies. Effectively leverage the strengths of the VA and IHS at the national and local levels to afford the delivery of optimal clinical care.	• Share specialty services • Develop joint credentialing and privileging of staff • Develop joint training initiatives • Develop and implement new models of care using new technologies, including telehealth services
2. Promote patient-centered collaboration and facilitate communication among VA, IHS, Native American veterans, tribal facilities, and Urban Indian Clinics.	• Establish mechanism to share electronic health records for patients receiving care in both systems and from tribally operated facilities • Improve the delivery of care through sharing of care processes, programs, and services (for example, post-traumatic stress disorder and diabetes management)
3. In consultation with tribes at the regional and local levels, establish effective partnerships and sharing agreements among VA headquarters and facilities, IHS headquarters and IHS, tribal, and Urban Indian Health programs in support of Native American veterans.	• Develop standard preapproved language for inclusion of one agency into the other agency's existing contracts • Develop preapproved templates for agreements to facilitate local, regional, and national collaboration
4. Ensure that appropriate resources are identified and available to support programs for Native American veterans.	• Develop payment and reimbursement policies and mechanisms for veterans receiving care in both systems
5. Improve health promotion and disease prevention services to Native Americans to address community-based wellness.	• Improve the delivery of care through sharing of care processes, programs, and services (for example, post-traumatic stress disorder and diabetes management)

Source: GAO analysis of information provided by VA and IHS.

Workgroups

VA and IHS created 12 workgroups tasked with responsibility for implementing and developing strategies to address the goals of the MOU, such as interoperability of health information technology; developing payment and reimbursement agreements; and sharing of care processes, programs, and services.[20] Each workgroup includes members from VA and IHS, a step that can foster mutual trust across diverse agency cultures and facilitate frequent communication across agencies to enhance shared understanding of collaboration goals, according to our previous work on interagency collaboration. According to VA and IHS officials, most of the workgroup members volunteered to serve on the workgroups and were self-selected, and VA officials told us that they have consulted with tribes on how to increase tribal participation in the workgroups. The agencies also told us that some workgroup members were asked to participate because of their subject-matter expertise.[21]

Table 2. Goals of Eight Workgroups Interviewed and Corresponding Department of Veterans Affairs (VA) / Indian Health Service (IHS) Memorandum of Understanding (MOU) Goals

Workgroup	Goals	Crosswalk to MOU goals
Coordination of Care	• Increase access to and quality of care. • Promote patient-centered collaboration and increase coordination of care, including comanagement of dual- eligible veterans. Work with tribal urban organizations.	Goal 1: Increase access to and improve quality of health care and services to the mutual benefit of both agencies. Goal 2: Promote patient- centered collaboration and facilitate communication.
Health Information Technology	• Improve care through the development of health information technology. • Establish system to share electronic health records.	Goal 1: Increase access to and improve quality of health care and services to the mutual benefit of both agencies. Goal 2: Promote patient-centered collaboration and facilitate communication.
System Level	• Plan and implement system-level resources to share information about contracts and purchasing arrangements.	Goal 3: Establish effective partnerships and sharing agreements. Goal 4: Ensure that appropriate resources are identified and available to support programs.
Payment and Reimbursement	• Design system to ensure VA and IHS systems are compatible for the billing and collecting process under contracts or agreements.	Goal 4: Ensure that appropriate resources are identified and available to support programs.
Sharing of Care Process, Programs and Services	• Several MOU goals, including improving access to and quality of care for post-traumatic stress disorder	Goal 1: Increase access to and improve quality of health care and services to the mutual benefit of both agencies.

Table 2. (Continued)

Workgroup	Goals	Crosswalk to MOU goals
	among Native American veterans. • Conduct outreach to tribal areas in areas such as public health and suicide prevention. • Develop and update suicide prevention training. • Provide IHS pharmacists access to VA programs to streamline pharmacy dispensing activities. Coordinate and collaborate to improve the lives of elderly and frail Native Americans, and increase access to VA's home-based primary care program.	Goal 2: Promote patient-centered collaboration and facilitate communication. Goal 3: Establish effective partnerships and sharing agreements. Goal 5: Improve health-promotion and disease-prevention services to Native Americans to address community-based wellness.
Training and Recruitment	• Increase capability and improve quality through training and workforce development, sharing of educational and training opportunities, and the development of joint training initiatives. • Increase access to care through sharing of staff and enhanced recruitment and retention of professional staff.	Goal 1: Increase access to and improve quality of health care and services to the mutual benefit of both agencies.
Alaska	• Increase access to services and benefits of IHS and VA. • Improve coordination of care, including comanagement, for Native American veterans served by both VA and tribal organizations. • Increase availability of services, in accordance with law, by the development of payment and reimbursement policies and mechanisms.	Goal 1: Increase access to and improve quality of health care and services to the mutual benefit of both agencies. Goal 2: Promote patient-centered collaboration and facilitate communication. Goal 3: Establish effective partnerships and sharing agreements Goal 4: Ensure that appropriate resources are identified and available to support programs. Goal 5: Improve health-promotion and disease-prevention services to Native

Workgroup	Goals	Crosswalk to MOU goals
		Americans to address community-based wellness.
Oversight	• Set priorities for the Joint Implementation Task Force to identify the strategies and plans for accomplishing the tasks and aims of the MOU, and help the task force follow the strategy and plans of the MOU. • Meet with and receive updates from other workgroups and elevate issues identified by the workgroups. • Develop reports on progress in implementing the MOU.	Goal 1: Increase access to and improve quality of health care and services to the mutual benefit of both agencies. Goal 2: Promote patient-centered collaboration and facilitate communication. Goal 3: Establish effective partnerships and sharing agreements. Goal 4: Ensure that appropriate resources are identified and available to support programs. Goal 5: Improve health-promotion and disease-prevention services to Native Americans to address community-based wellness.

Source: GAO evaluation of interviews with workgroups and agency officials and the MOU.

Goals established by each workgroup appear to be aligned with MOU goals. Specifically, all eight of the workgroups we interviewed described goals that were consistent with the MOU goals.[22] Table 2 lists each workgroup we interviewed and provides a crosswalk between workgroup goals and the corresponding MOU goal or strategy.

Joint Implementation Task Force

VA and IHS created the Joint Implementation Task Force to oversee the overall implementation of the MOU. This task force comprises officials from both agencies including from the Office of the Secretary of Veterans Affairs, the IHS Chief Medical Officer, and the director of VA's Office of Tribal Government Relations, and is scheduled to meet quarterly. It develops implementation policy and procedures for policy-related issues identified by the workgroups; creates performance metrics and timelines, evaluates progress; and compiles an annual report on progress in MOU implementation. Creating a mechanism, such as a task force, intended not only to address issues arising from potential incompatibility of standards and policies across agencies but also to monitor, evaluate, and report on MOU results, can help to facilitate collaboration, according to our previous work on interagency collaboration.

Table 3. GAO Evaluation of Performance Metrics and Measures Developed to Monitor Progress toward Department of Veterans Affairs (VA) / Indian Health Service (IHS) Memorandum of Understanding (MOU) Goals

Metric	Measures	GAO evaluation
Metric 1: Programs increased or enhanced as a result of the VA-IHS MOU	1. Number of programs enhanced and increased 2. Number of events and activities to increase or enhance the programs 3. Number of veterans impacted 4. Met purposes of MOU (yes or no) 5. Met intent of MOU (yes or no) 6. Level of VA-IHS-Tribal participation (poor, fair, good, excellent)	Inadequate Tangible and measurable, but not clearly aligned with an MOU goal and would not allow agencies to determine how well MOU goals are achieved.
Metric 2: Outreach activities that are the result of MOU partnerships	1. Types of outreach events held 2. Number of outreach events held 3. Number of veterans and others (families, caregivers) impacted 4. Met purposes of MOU (yes or no) 5. Met intent of MOU (yes or no) 6. Level of VA-IHS-Tribal participation (poor, fair, good, excellent)	Inadequate Tangible and measurable but not clearly aligned with an MOU goal, and would not allow agencies to determine how well MOU goals are achieved.
Metric 3: Development of reimbursement agreements and sharing agreements as a result of the MOU	1. Number of sharing agreements developed 2. Number of tribes impacted 3. Number of reimbursement agreements developed 4. Number of tribes impacted 5. Met purposes of MOU (yes or no) 6. Met intent of MOU (yes or no) 7. Level of VA-IHS-Tribal participation (poor, fair, good, excellent)	Adequate Tangible and measureable, aligned with an MOU goal, and allows the agencies to measure progress toward goals three and four.

Source: GAO analysis of information provided by VA and IHS.

Note: The five MOU goals are:

(1) Increase access to and improve quality of health care and services to the mutual benefit of both agencies. Effectively leverage the strengths of the VA and IHS at the national and local levels to afford the delivery of optimal clinical care.
(2) Promote patient-centered collaboration and facilitate communication among VA, IHS, Native American veterans, tribal facilities, and Urban Indian Clinics.
(3) In consultation with tribes at the regional and local levels, establish effective partnerships and sharing agreements among VA headquarters and facilities, IHS headquarters and IHS, tribal, and Urban Indian Health programs in support of Native American veterans.
(4) Ensure that appropriate resources are identified and available to support programs for Native American veterans.
(5) Improve health promotion and disease prevention services to Native Americans to address community-based wellness.

VA and IHS Performance Metrics Do Not Adequately Measure Progress on the MOU Goals

The process developed by the Joint Implementation Task Force to monitor the implementation of the MOU includes obtaining data on three performance metrics; however, two of the three metrics do not allow the agencies to measure progress toward the MOU's goals. Our previous work has found that successful performance metrics should be tangible and measureable, clearly aligned with specific goals, and demonstrate the degree to which desired results are achieved.[23] Although all three of the performance metrics are tangible and measurable, only one is also clearly aligned with a specific goal and defined in a manner that would allow the agencies to adequately measure the degree to which desired results are achieved. The other two metrics are inadequate because their connection to a specific goal is not clear and they lack qualitative measures that would allow the agencies to measure the degree to which desired results are achieved. For example, one MOU goal is to increase access to and improve quality of health care services, but none of the metrics mention any targets specifically linked to increased access or improved quality of care. Another goal is to establish effective partnerships and sharing agreements among the agencies and the tribes in support of Native American veterans. Although one of the metrics appears to be related to this goal, in that it is focused on measuring the number of outreach activities that are a result of partnerships, it lacks measures to determine how well the outreach activities are meeting the goal of establishing effective partnerships or other potential goals to which the outreach may contribute, such as facilitating communication among VA, IHS, veterans, and tribally operated facilities. The metrics would therefore not enable VA and IHS to determine how well these specific goals are being achieved. Table 3 describes the performance metrics and performance measures and our evaluation of them.

Using these metrics, the agencies have issued MOU progress reports, but the metrics included in the reports generally are not clearly tied specifically to the goals of the MOU, nor do they allow the agencies to determine how well MOU goals have been achieved. Leading public- sector organizations have found that metrics that are clearly linked to goals and allow determination of how well goals are achieved are key steps to becoming more results-oriented. For example:

- According to the agencies' fiscal year 2011-2012 metrics report,[24] for Metric 1 (programs increased or enhanced as a result of the MOU), more than 15 programs were enhanced or increased as the result of the MOU, and 440 events and activities occurred that increased or enhanced the programs. The report then provides examples of programs that have been enhanced, such as a care coordination program in which a registered nurse "works with Indian Health, Tribal Programs, and other agencies and hospitals through direct meetings at various facilities to ensure communication and improved care." However, the report does not always describe information that would allow the agencies to determine how well each activity contributes to meeting MOU goals. For instance, in the description of an enhanced care coordination program noted above, the report does not indicate how the agencies determined that communication has improved among participants. Absent this information, it is not clear how the agencies could draw conclusions about whether improved communication has actually been facilitated and therefore how well the activity contributed to meeting the MOU goal of promoting patient- centered collaboration and facilitating communication.
- According to the metrics report, for Metric 2 (outreach activities increased or enhanced as a result of MOU partnerships), eight types of activities were increased or enhanced. However, the report lists only seven types of outreach and does not include enough information to determine how well the outreach contributes to meeting MOU goals. For example, one outreach activity cited in the report, "Outreach to promote implementation of new technologies," includes the activity

"VA Office of Telehealth Services (OTS) Coordinator participated in Web-ex sessions with IHS on use of technology to improve patient care." Although not stated in the report, this activity appears to help implement the MOU strategy of enhancing access through the development and implementation of new models of care using new technologies, including telehealth, related to the MOU goals of promoting patient-centered care and increasing access to care. However, while outreach activities are measurable and tangible, and might help to achieve goals of the MOU, the report does not state how the agencies will determine whether the sessions actually were effective in improving patient care or increasing access, information that is necessary to allow the agencies to tell how well the activity helps achieve the MOU goals.

- For each metric, the agencies report whether the activities "met the purpose of the MOU," "met the intent of the MOU," and whether the "level of VA-IHS-Tribal participation" was poor, fair, good, or excellent. While determining whether the agencies' activities meet the purpose and intent of the MOU is a critical step, and obtaining tribal participation is consistent with MOU goals, the report does not describe how these determinations were made. Agency officials told us that these determinations were made subjectively by each workgroup while keeping in mind the goals and strategies in the MOU.

The weaknesses we found in these performance metrics could limit the ability of VA and IHS managers to gauge progress and make decisions about whether to expand or modify programs or activities, because the agencies will not have information on how well programs are supporting MOU goals. VA and IHS officials told us that they developed these performance metrics because the initial performance metrics, drafted by the workgroups themselves and other VA and IHS staff, varied in quality. The three metrics and measures were intended to provide some simple, measurable ways for workgroups to report on their progress. However, they also acknowledged that there were weaknesses in the measures and told us that refining these performance metrics is a priority. According to the officials, they plan to revise workgroup metrics by April 2013 and on a continuous basis going forward. In doing so, they plan to consult subject-matter experts and existing VA and IHS performance metrics, for example, prevention of hospital admissions in home-based primary care programs.

VA and IHS Lack Effective Processes to Overcome the Challenges of Consulting with a Large Number of Diverse, Sovereign Tribes

Mainly because of the large number of diverse tribal communities and tribal sovereignty, VA and IHS face unique challenges associated with coordinating and communicating to implement the MOU. VA and IHS have processes in place for consulting with tribes, but these measures fall short in several respects and do not ensure such consultation is effective.

VA and IHS Face Challenges Implementing the MOU Related to the Large Number of Diverse, Sovereign Tribes

VA and IHS officials told us the large number (566) of federally recognized tribes and differing customs and policy-making structures present logistical challenges in widespread implementation of the MOU within tribal communities.[25] For instance, according to some VA officials, in some tribes as a matter of protocol, an agency must be invited on tribal lands or be sponsored by a council member in order to address a tribal council. Such a policy could add administrative processes that might delay implementation and require greater sensitivity from agency officials, adding to the challenge of consulting with tribes. As another example, the title or position of the tribal person designated to make decisions regarding health care may differ from tribe to tribe, complicating the decision-making process among VA, IHS, and tribes. VA officials told us in some tribes, for example, a tribal leader may have several roles, only one of which is making decisions on health care, whereas in other tribes there may be a tribal health director whom the tribal leader has designated to manage health care in the tribal community. Potentially, these differences can affect the speed and degree at which collective decisions can be made.

In addition, VA and IHS officials noted that tribal sovereignty further adds to the logistical complexity of the efforts of the agencies to implement the MOU. Tribal sovereignty includes the inherent right to govern and protect the health, safety, and welfare of tribal members. Indian tribes have a legal and political government-to-government relationship with the federal government, meaning federal agencies interact with tribes as governments, not as special interest groups or individuals. VA and IHS officials told us that because of tribal sovereignty, tribally operated facilities may choose whether or not to participate in a particular opportunity for collaboration related to the MOU, which makes it challenging to achieve some of the goals of the MOU. VA and IHS can inform tribes of an opportunity but cannot require them to participate. For example:

- In order to meet the MOU goal to establish standard mechanisms for access to electronic health record (EHR) information for shared patients, VA and IHS have coordinated to adapt their information technology systems to allow them both to participate in the eHealth Exchange, a national effort led by the Department of Health and Human Services for sharing EHR information.[26] However, EHR workgroup members told us that some tribally operated facilities have opted to use an off-the-shelf product in place of the IHS system, which the workgroup members do not have the resources to support.
- In another instance, as a part of their efforts to meet the MOU goal to establish effective partnerships and sharing agreements, VA and IHS are working to implement VA's Consolidated Mail Outpatient Pharmacy (CMOP) throughout IHS. Workgroup members assigned to these activities said they plan to implement the program in all IHS-operated facilities by spring 2013 but cannot require tribally operated facilities to participate. Some smaller tribal communities with more limited postal access are not interested in using the CMOP program, according to the workgroup members.

VA and IHS Processes in Place to Overcome the Complexities Associated with Consulting with Tribes Do Not Always Ensure Effective Consultation

VA and IHS communicate MOU-related information with the tribes through written correspondence, in-person meetings, and other steps, as is consistent with internal controls calling for effective external communications with groups that can have a serious effect on programs and other activities; however, according to tribal stakeholders we interviewed, these methods for consultation have not always met the needs of the tribal communities, and the agencies have acknowledged that effective consultation has been challenging.

Written Correspondence

VA and IHS send written correspondence (known as "Dear Tribal Leader" letters) regarding the MOU to tribal communities. However, the agencies have acknowledged that because of the large and diverse nature of the tribes, they have struggled to reach the tribal member designated to make health care decisions with information about the MOU. Both VA officials and members of tribal communities told us that, because tribal leaders are not always the tribal person designated to make decisions regarding health care, the "Dear Tribal Leader" letters may not always make their way to tribal members designated to take action on health care matters. VA officials told us that their formal consultation is conducted with tribal leaders. However, these officials also noted that, in addition to the letters sent to tribal leaders, they have a network of contacts within each tribe that includes, among others, tribal health directors, and this network receives concurrent notice of communication with tribal leaders via conference calls, listservs, and newsletters. IHS officials said sometimes, in addition to the tribal leader, they may also send letters to, or otherwise communicate directly with, tribal health program directors if they know of them. However, they also noted they do not maintain a specific record— such as a listserv—of tribal health program directors. Without reaching the tribal members responsible for decision-making on healthcare matters, VA and IHS may not always be effectively communicating with tribes about the status of the MOU and its related activities nor be obtaining tribal feedback that is critical with respect to implementation of the MOU.

Likewise, seven tribal stakeholders we spoke with noted similar concerns regarding the "Dear Tribal Leader" letters as VA and IHS. For example, one tribal stakeholder said letters should go to a specific person, such as a tribal health director, to ensure that the information is seen by the right people in a timely manner. It may take the tribes time to pass along letters sent only to tribal leaders to the tribal health director or other appropriate people, by which point any deadlines included in the correspondence could be missed. Once the information has reached the tribal leader, tribes bear the responsibility to ensure it is passed on to the appropriate audience in a timely manner.

Another specific concern tribal stakeholders that we spoke with expressed relating to written correspondence was that the agencies sometimes use the letters to simply inform them of steps the agencies have taken without consulting the tribes, as called for by the agencies' tribal consultation policies. For example, some tribal stakeholders said VA and IHS did not include them in the original development of the 2010 MOU, even though the goals and activities in the MOU could directly affect them. According to 10 of the tribal stakeholders we spoke with, tribes should have been included in developing the MOU, which addresses proposed plans, policies, and programmatic actions that may affect tribes. For example, the MOU seeks to improve delivery of health care by developing and implementing new models of care using new technologies, including telehealth services such as telepsychiatry. Instead, the agencies solicited tribal comments after the agencies had signed the MOU. According to two tribal stakeholders, the agencies were not responsive to the comments provided on the MOU. One stakeholder said their comments were not acknowledged upon receipt nor did IHS ever follow up on the issues raised by their comments. The stakeholder suggested IHS designate a point person to track feedback and ensure follow-up. VA and IHS officials told us that they did not hold tribal consultation meetings before the signing of the MOU because they viewed the MOU as an agency-to-agency agreement rather than as an agreement between the agencies and the various tribes.

In-person Meetings

VA and IHS officials said they hold quarterly meetings with tribal communities and also attend events, such as conferences held by Native American interest organizations. Three tribal stakeholders told us that when the agencies have held consultation meetings, the meetings are not interactive enough—stating that agency officials speak for the majority of the time—and that VA does not provide enough information prior to these meetings. These tribal stakeholders said providing information ahead of time could allow tribes to better prepare for meetings, discuss issues as a tribe beforehand, and determine which tribal members should attend. If tribal officials with the authority and desire to work with VA and IHS do not receive needed information on opportunities because of an ineffective consultation process, local facility leadership may not have readily available access to information necessary to examine which collaborative opportunities are present, and thus VA and IHS may be hindered in their efforts to coordinate health care for Native American veterans.

VA and IHS are undertaking other efforts designed to enhance consultation with tribes. These include the following steps:

- In January 2011, VA established the Office of Tribal Government Relations (OTGR) to serve as the point of contact for tribes. According to VA officials, this office conducted four consultation meetings in 2012 and employed five field staff to help manage communication with tribal communities and to work with IHS on local MOU implementation efforts.

- In February 2011, VA released the agency's tribal consultation policy. VA officials said they are developing a report that will explain the process for evaluating comments from tribes and making decisions based on them. The officials expect the report to be released to the public in the spring of 2013.
- The agencies have made more local efforts to communicate with tribes, which have led to some success. For example, agency officials and tribal stakeholders noted that the workgroup assigned to implement MOU activities in Alaska used successful methods for working with tribes. The Alaska workgroup told us they cultivated a relationship with an Alaskan tribal health organization in order to get advice on the appropriate customs for consulting with individual tribes there. In addition, the workgroup said they scheduled consultation meetings in conjunction with other meetings, which would limit the amount of travel tribal community members would need to undertake. VA employees also took cultural awareness training, and VA officials visited Alaska to demonstrate the agency's dedication to providing care to Native American veterans, which, according to the workgroup, led to buy-in from tribal communities. VA and Alaskan tribes have signed 26 reimbursement agreements.

Some tribal stakeholders that we spoke with have acknowledged the steps taken by the agencies thus far as positive but in some cases expressed concerns regarding tribal consultation. In the case of the tribes working with the Alaska workgroup, one stakeholder praised VA's efforts to work with tribal health organizations to communicate with tribes. In another example, two tribal stakeholders said they approved of OTGR's establishment as an office dedicated to Native American veterans' issues. However, four tribal stakeholders expressed concerns that, despite the creation of OTGR, VA still has not always been effective in its efforts to consult with tribes or be responsive to tribal input provided during consultation. For example, one stakeholder questioned whether consultation was done with every tribe and described VA's consultation process as sporadic. This stakeholder's concern implies that VA's outreach efforts may not be systematically reaching all tribal communities. However, VA officials told us that, in addition to issuing notices in the Federal Register and Dear Tribal Leader letters, they have a systematic process of hosting training summits for tribes and scheduling regular conference calls and presentations to tribal leadership. In another instance, one tribal community member said OTGR lacks—and thus cannot disperse to tribes—the technical knowledge necessary for tribes to partner with VA on activities such as negotiating reimbursement agreements. VA officials noted that OTGR staff may not always be technical experts on a given topic but said they are able to identify those experts and play a key role in linking tribes with them.

CONCLUSION

Coordination between VA and IHS is essential to ensuring that high-quality health care is provided to dually eligible Native American veterans. While the 2010 MOU includes common goals that should facilitate agency coordination, and the agencies have created workgroups tasked to implement the MOU, we found that a critical mechanism for monitoring the implementation of the MOU, the agreement's performance metrics, has weaknesses. Specifically, the inadequacies we found in performance metrics could limit the agencies' ability to measure progress towards MOU goals and ultimately make decisions about programs or activities.

Overcoming the challenges related to working with a large number of diverse, sovereign tribes is also essential to successfully achieving the goals of the MOU. Although steps have been taken to consult with tribes regarding the MOU and related activities, consultation has not always been effective in assuring that the people designated to make health care decisions in each tribe are reached and tribes are included in planning and implementation efforts. Ineffective consultation with tribal communities could delay or limit potential VA, IHS, and tribal community partnerships to achieve the goals of the MOU and could hinder agency efforts to gain support for MOU activities and address the health care needs of Native American veterans.

RECOMMENDATIONS FOR EXECUTIVE ACTION

To ensure the health care needs of Native American veterans are addressed most efficiently and effectively, we recommend that the Secretary of Veterans Affairs and Secretary of Health and Human Services take the following two actions:

- As the agencies move forward with revising the MOU's performance metrics and measures, ensure that the revised metrics and measures allow decision makers to gauge whether achievement of the metrics and measures supports attainment of MOU goals.
- Develop processes to better ensure that consultation with tribes is effective, including the following:
  - A process to identify the appropriate tribal members with whom to communicate MOU-related information, which should include methods for keeping such identification up-to-date.
  - A process to clearly outline and communicate to tribal communities the agencies' response to tribal input, including any changes in policies and programs or other effects that result from incorporating tribal input.
  - A process to establish timelines for releasing information to tribal communities to ensure they have enough time to review and provide input or, in the case of meetings, determine the appropriate tribal member to attend the event.

AGENCY COMMENTS

We provided draft copies of this report to VA and the Department of Health and Human Services for review. Both agencies concurred with our recommendations. In addition, VA provided us with comments on the draft report, as well as general and technical comments, which were incorporated in the draft as appropriate.

Randall Williamson
Director, Health Care

End Notes

[1] According to the U.S. Census Bureau, in 2011 approximately 150,000 individuals identified themselves as Native American veterans. This includes only individuals who identified as American Indian or Alaska Native alone and not in combination with another racial group. Therefore, it likely underestimates the number of Native American veterans.

[2] *Oversight Hearing on Programs and Services for Native Veterans*: hearing before the Committee on Indian Affairs, United States Senate, 112th Cong (May 24, 2012).

[3] S. Rep. No. 112-168, at 45 (May 22, 2012).

[4] VA is required to reimburse federally and tribally operated facilities for health care services provided to beneficiaries who are eligible for such services from VA. 25 U.S.C. § 1645(c).

[5] The eight workgroups we interviewed were: (1) Coordination of Care; (2) Health Information Technology; (3) System Level; (4) Payment and Reimbursement; (5) Sharing of Care Process, Programs and Services; (6) Training and Recruitment; (7) Oversight; and (8) Alaska. VA and IHS count the Training and Recruitment Workgroup as two separate workgroups. However, because these two workgroups share similar goals, an IHS official told us they combined them into one workgroup, and for the purposes of this report we considered them as one workgroup. There are also four other workgroups covering: (1) Services and Benefits, (2) New Technologies; (3) Cultural Competency and Awareness; and (4) Emergency and Disaster Preparedness. We did not interview these workgroups because they did not directly relate to our objectives.

[6] GAO, *Results-Oriented Government: Practices That Can Help Enhance and Sustain Collaboration among Federal Agencies*, GAO-06-15 (Washington, D.C.: Oct. 21, 2005); *Managing for Results: Key Considerations for Implementing Interagency Collaborative Mechanisms*, GAO-12-1022 (Washington, D.C.: Sept. 27, 2012); *Executive Guide: Effectively Implementing the Government Performance and Results Act*, GAO/GGD-96-118 (Washington, D.C.: June 1996); and *Agencies' Strategic Plans Under GPRA: Key Questions to Facilitate Congressional Review*, GAO/GGD-10.1.16 (Washington, D.C.: May 1997).

[7] GAO, *Internal Control Standards: Internal Control Management and Evaluation Tool*, GAO-01-1008G (Washington, D.C.: August 2001).

[8] For more information on federal funding for non–federally recognized tribes, see GAO, *Indian Issues: Federal Funding for Non-Federally Recognized Tribes*, GAO-12-348 (Washington, D.C.: Apr. 12, 2012).

[9] To be eligible for IHS health care services, an individual must be closely affiliated with a federally recognized tribe, as evidenced by such factors as membership; enrollment; residence on tax-exempt land; ownership of restricted property; active participation in tribal affairs; or other relevant factors indicative of Native American descent. See 42 C.F.R. § 136.12.

[10] To manage its provision of health care services for eligible veterans, VA operates a system of annual patient enrollment in accordance with eight listed priorities. See 38 U.S.C. § 1705.

[11] Under the Indian Self-Determination and Education Assistance Act, as amended, federally recognized tribes can enter into self-determination contracts or self-governance compacts with the Secretary of Health and Human Services to take over administration of IHS programs for Native Americans previously administered by IHS on their behalf because of their status as Indians. Self-governance compacts allow tribes to consolidate and assume administration of all programs, services, activities, and competitive grants administered throughout IHS, or portions thereof, that are carried out for the benefit of Native Americans because of their status as Indians. Self determination contracts allow tribes to assume administration of a program, programs, or portions thereof. See 25 U.S.C. §§ 450f(a) (self-determination contracts)and 458aaa-4(b)(1) (self-governance compacts).

[12] Federal agencies are required to consult with Alaska Native corporations on the same basis as Indian tribes under Executive Order 13175. Pub. L. No. 108-199, div. H, § 161, 118 Stat. 3, 452 (2004), as amended.

[13] See 74 Fed. Reg. 57,881 (Nov. 9, 2009).

[14] According to the policy, the principal focus of consultation is the tribally designated "tribal official" and that consultation will be initiated by means of written notification.

[15] GAO-06-15 and GAO-12-1022.

[16] GAO-12-1022.

[17] GAO/GGD-10.1.16 and GAO/GGD-96-118 (for this report, GAO studied a number of leading public-sector organizations that were successfully becoming more results- oriented,

including state governments such as in Florida, Texas, and Virginia; and foreign governments such as in Australia and the United Kingdom).

[18] GAO-01-1008G.

[19] GAO-12-1022.

[20] The 12 workgroups are: (1) Coordination of Care; (2) Health Information Technology; (3) System Level; (4) Payment and Reimbursement; (5) Sharing of Care Process, Programs and Services; (6) Training and Recruitment; (7) Oversight; (8) Alaska; (9) Services and Benefits; (10) New Technologies; (11) Cultural Competency and Awareness; and (12) Emergency and Disaster Preparedness.

[21] The officials told us that in cases where a workgroup lacks authority to implement an MOU task, workgroup members would notify MOU coordinators designated by each agency, who would then notify the appropriate agency officials about the issue.

[22] We did not interview 4 workgroups because they did not directly relate to our objectives: (1) Services and Benefits; (2) New Technologies; (3) Cultural Competency and Awareness; and (4) Emergency and Disaster Preparedness.

[23] GAO/GGD-96-118 and GAO/GGD-10.1.16.

[24] Department of Veterans Affairs and Indian Health Service, *Department of Veterans Affairs (VA) Indian Health Service (IHS) Memorandum of Understanding (MOU) Metrics Report—Fiscal Year (FY) 2011/2012.*

[25] In addition to the federally recognized tribes, there are more than 400 non–federally recognized tribes. Although these non–federally recognized tribes may not receive IHS funding and members may not be eligible for IHS services, VA has an obligation to serve their members who are eligible for VA services.

[26] The eHealth Exchange is a set of standards, services, and policies that enable the secure exchange of health information over the Internet.

In: Veterans
Editor: Timothy C. Roberts

ISBN: 978-1-63117-046-1

Chapter 3

EMPLOYMENT FOR VETERANS: TRENDS AND PROGRAMS*

Benjamin Collins, David H. Bradley, Robert Jay Dilger, Cassandria Dortch, Lawrence Kapp, Sean Lowry and Christine Scott

SUMMARY

Veterans' employment outcomes in the civilian labor market are an issue of ongoing congressional interest. This report offers introductory data on veterans' performance in the civilian labor market as well as a discussion of veteran-targeted federal programs that provide employment-related benefits and services.

According to federal data, the unemployment rate for veterans who served after September 2001 is higher than the unemployment rate for nonveterans. Conversely, the unemployment rate for veterans from prior service periods (a much larger population than post-9/11 veterans) is lower than the nonveteran unemployment rate. The varied demographic factors of each of these populations likely contribute to these variations, though their degree of influence is unclear.

---

* This is an edited, reformatted and augmented version of a Congressional Research Service publication, CRS Report for Congress R42790, dated January 10, 2013.

There are a number of federal programs to assist veterans in developing job skills and securing civilian employment. Broadly speaking, these programs can be divided into (1) general veterans' programs, (2) programs that target veterans with service-connected disabilities, and (3) competitive grant programs that offer supplemental services but may be limited in scope.

General veterans' programs begin with transition programs that are provided to exiting members of the Armed Forces. These transition programs cover a variety of topics including information on identifying occupations that align with military skills and specializations, conducting job searches, applying for employment, and navigating veterans' benefits. One of the most common veterans' benefits is educational funding through the GI Bill. The GI Bill programs typically provide funding for tuition, fees, housing, books and supplies, and other educational costs while the veteran is enrolled. Veterans who are no longer eligible for the GI Bill may receive training benefits through the Veterans Retraining Assistance Program (VRAP).

Veterans who are seeking employment without obtaining additional training may receive job search assistance and other services from Local Veterans Employment Representatives (LVER). Veterans who wish to pursue employment in the federal government are assisted by several policies that give them preference in the competitive hiring process or, in some cases, allow them to forego the competitive process and be appointed directly. Veterans who wish to start a small business may receive loans and technical assistance from the Small Business Administration (SBA).

Veterans with service-connected disabilities who have obstacles to employment may be assisted by the Vocational Rehabilitation and Employment (VR&E) program. This program provides assistance in identifying an occupation that is consistent with the veterans' skills and interests and providing the services (including educational services) necessary to achieve that outcome. Disabled veterans can also receive assistance from the Disabled Veterans Outreach Program (DVOP), which provides assistance in local labor markets.

In addition to these nationwide programs, the federal government also funds competitive grant programs for state, local, and private entities to provide employment-oriented services to veterans. These include the Veterans Workforce Investment Program (VWIP), which may provide training or employment services and Veterans Upward Bound (VUB), which prepares educationally disadvantaged veterans for postsecondary coursework.

BACKGROUND

Veterans' employment outcomes in the civilian sector are an issue of ongoing congressional interest that has received particular attention during the current period of relatively high unemployment. A number of programs currently exist to assist veterans in obtaining or training for civilian employment. There is regular congressional debate about expanding or otherwise amending these programs to better serve veterans.

This report discusses veterans' employment trends and programs. The first section presents data on veterans' employment outcomes, identifying recent trends, and discussing issues to consider when interpreting veterans' employment data. The following sections present brief discussions of existing programs that provide employment-related services to veterans. These services are divided into (1) general programs that are broadly available to veterans, (2) programs that target veterans with service-connected disabilities, and (3) competitive grant programs that provide additional employment-related services to veterans but may be limited in scope or availability.

Notably, this report does not attempt to provide an exhaustive list of all programs that may assist veterans in the labor market nor does it attempt to provide comprehensive information on the programs is discusses. Instead, it aims to provide a broad overview of the largest employment- related programs as well as other initiatives that may inform future policy. For detailed information on each program, readers are encouraged to refer to the CRS reports or other sources that are referenced in each section.[1]

EMPLOYMENT TRENDS AMONG VETERANS[2]

Estimates of veterans' employment and unemployment are published by the Bureau of Labor Statistics (BLS). The estimates are derived from the Current Population Survey (CPS), a monthly household survey in which respondents may self-identify as veterans. Veterans' employment outcomes are frequently compared to the employment outcomes of nonveterans to establish veterans' relative performance in the labor market.

This section will divide workers into three groups: (1) Gulf War II veterans who served at any point after September 2001, (2) veterans from prior service periods, and (3) nonveterans.[3] Since these populations vary in many characteristics that may influence employment outcomes, comparisons between these groups should be conducted with caution.

Recent employment outcomes for veterans and non-veterans are presented in **Table 1**.[4] As the table shows, the unemployment rate for Gulf War II (GWII) veterans is higher than the unemployment rates of both veterans from other periods of service as well as nonveterans. GWII veterans, however, constitute less than 20% of the veteran labor force (about 2 million of just under 11 million).

Several factors that are not observable in **Table 1** should also be considered when interpreting the employment data in the table.[5]

- *The GWII veteran labor force is younger than the nonveteran labor force.* About 63% of GWII veterans in the labor force are under the age of 35, compared to about 37% of nonveterans in the labor force. Since younger workers generally have higher unemployment rates than older workers, GWII veterans' relative youth may influence their unemployment rate.[6]
- *Veterans have a different educational distribution than nonveterans.* Among those in the labor force, only 1% of GWII veterans and 3% of other veterans have less than a high school education, compared to 9% of nonveterans. Conversely, the proportion of college graduates among the labor forces of GWII veterans (31%) and other veterans (30%) are somewhat lower than nonveterans (36%).[7] The effect of this different educational distribution on veterans' employment outcomes is unclear.
- *Disability issues.* In 2011, approximately 14% of all veterans and 26% of GWII veterans reported a service-connected disability. While service-connected disabilities do appear to be related to lower rates of labor force participation and higher rates of unemployment among labor force participants, the differences in employment outcomes between disabled and non-disabled veterans are modest. Among veterans of all service periods, the labor force participation rate for veterans with a service-connected disability was slightly lower than for veterans without a service-connected disability (49% v. 52%) and the unemployment rate was slightly higher (8.5% v. 7.9%). When limited to GWII veterans, the difference in participation rate is similar (80% v. 84%) and difference in unemployment rate (12.1% and 9.5%) is somewhat larger.[8] Comparable data on employment outcomes for nonveterans with disabilities are not available.

- *Categorization of post-military transition period.* Recent veterans who have not yet secured post-service employment are categorized as unemployed and entitled to unemployment insurance. The classification of this transition period may increase GWII veterans' unemployment rate.

Figure 1 presents recent historical data on unemployment rates for GWII veterans, other veterans, and nonveterans.[9] Several trends emerge over the 17-quarter reference period:

- *The unemployment rate for GWII veterans is very dynamic.*[10] This is likely due to their relatively small sample size in the CPS. Short-term trends for this population (such as the spike in the unemployment rate in mid-2010 and the large drop in the unemployment rate at the beginning on 2012) should be interpreted with caution.
- *The unemployment rate for GWII veterans is typically above that of other veterans and nonveterans.* The 17-quarter average unemployment rate was 10.7% among GWII veterans, 7.4% among other veterans, and 8.7% among nonveterans.
  Quarterly data are not available prior to the fourth quarter of 2008. Annual data from 2005 to 2008, however, are similar to recent trends with unemployment rates for GWII veterans that are higher than those of nonveterans and unemployment rates of other veterans that are lower than those of nonveterans.[11]

Table 1. Employment Outcomes by Veteran Status, Fourth Quarter 2012

	Population (thousands)	Labor Force (thousands)	Unemployed (thousands)	Unemployment Rate
All Veterans	**21,059**	**10,892**	**723**	**6.6%**
Gulf War II Veterans	2,544	2,101	215	10.2%
Other Veterans	18,514	8,791	507	5.8%
Nonveterans	**214,114**	**142,503**	**10,487**	**7.4%**

Source: Quarterly data calculated by CRS based on monthly data from the Bureau of Labor Statistics' Employment Situation historical data for Table A-5, generated at http://www.bls.gov/webapps/legacy/ cpsatab5.htm.

Notes: Sum of veterans groups may not equal veterans total due to rounding. Gulf War II veterans are those who served any time after September 2001. Nonveterans exclude persons under age 18. Data are not seasonally adjusted; seasonally adjusted estimates are not available.

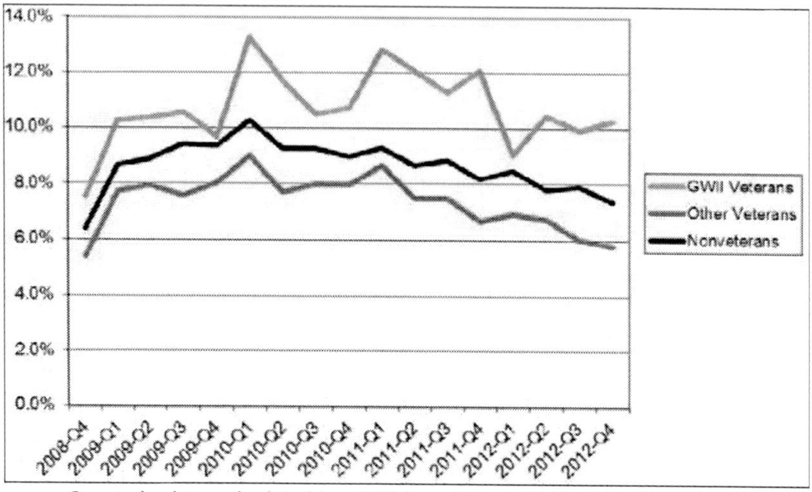

Source: Quarterly data calculated by CRS based on monthly data from the Bureau of Labor Statistics' Employment Situation historical data for Table A-5, generated at http://www.bls.gov/webapps/legacy/ cpsatab5.htm.

Notes: Gulf War II veterans are those who served any time after September 2001. Nonveterans excludes persons under age 18. Data are not seasonally adjusted so quarter-to-quarter comparisons should be conducted with caution. Seasonally adjusted estimates for veterans' employment are not available.

Figure 1. Unemployment Rates by Veteran Status, 2008-2012.

- *The unemployment rate for each group trends similarly over the reference period.* While the dynamic nature of the GWII veterans' unemployment rate somewhat masks this trend, each group's unemployment rate followed a generally upward trend from late 2008 to early 2010 and then a downward trend in the subsequent quarters. The similarity of these trends underscores the influence of the broader labor market on veterans' employment outcomes.

CURRENT EMPLOYMENT-RELATED PROGRAMS FOR VETERANS

This report highlights the primary training and employment services programs that are available to veterans. It does not, however, attempt to present a comprehensive list of employment-related programs for veterans. This report emphasizes programs available to veterans of active duty and generally omits discussion of programs that target former members of the military reserve. It also omits discussions of programs or program components that provide benefits to eligible family members of veterans.

The veteran-targeted programs in this report are presented in **Table 2**. Each is discussed in greater detail in the subsequent text. These programs are grouped into three categories:

- *Programs that are broadly available to veterans.* While they may have some eligibility limitations, these programs are generally available to veterans with or without a service-connected disability;
- *Programs that are available to veterans with service-connected disabilities.* These programs include the Vocational Rehabilitation and Employment program as well specialized versions of some generally available veterans programs; and
- *Competitive grant programs.* These programs fund employment-related services for veterans but may be limited in scope or local availability.

Table 2. Employment-Related Programs, Benefits, and Services for Veterans

Program	Description	FY2012 Funding
General Programs, Benefits, and Services for Veterans		
Transition Assistance Program (TAP) / Transition Goals Plans Success (Transition GPS)	TAP provides services to exiting service members related to obtaining civilian employment and otherwise transitioning to civilian life. Transition GPS is currently in the process of replacing TAP. Transition GPS will be a mandatory program for nearly all exiting service members with expanded services over a five-day curriculum.	$9 million appropriation from the Department of Labor (DOL); $6 million from the Department of Veterans Affairs (VA); $50 million from the Department of Defense (DOD)[a]
Educational Benefits (GI Bill)	GI Bill programs generally provide funds for educational costs as well as living expenses while enrolled in educational programs. The most-used program for recent veterans is the Post-9/11 GI Bill.	$10.5 billion[b]

Table 2. (Continued)

Program	Description	FY2012 Funding
Veterans Retraining Assistance Program (VRAP)	VRAP provides educational benefits for unemployed veterans between the ages of 35 and 60 who are not eligible for a GI Bill or other VA educational program. VRAP benefits are limited to 12 months.	$197 million[c]
Local Veterans Employment Representatives (LVER)	LVER funds state personnel positions that assist veterans in securing employment in their local area. LVER activities include but are not limited to outreach to local employers and referral to training or education benefits, LVER is funded out of Jobs for Veterans State Grant (JVSG) funds.	$165 million appropriation from DOL (also funds DVOP)
Federal Hiring Preferences and Special Hiring Authorities	Veterans receive preference when applying for nearly all competitively-hired federal employment. There are also special hiring authorities in which qualified veterans may be directly appointed to a position that would otherwise be competitively hired.	not applicable
Work Opportunity Tax Credit (WOTC)	Employers who hire veterans who meet various criteria (such as long-term unemployment or receipt of benefits under the Supplemental Nutrition Assistance Program) are eligible for a tax credit equal to a portion of the veteran's wages.	estimates limited to veteran provisions not available
Priority of Service in DOL training programs	Veterans receive priority of service for any DOL- funded training or employment service program that they are eligible for as a member of the general public.	not applicable
Small Business Administration (SBA) Programs	SBA has a variety of programs to assist veterans with developing and managing a small business, financing a small business, and acquiring federal contracts.	funding limited to veteran programs not available[e]
Programs for Veterans with Service-Connected Disabilities		
Vocational Rehabilitation and Employment (VR&E)	VR&E provides counseling to assist veterans with service-connected disabilities to identify an employment objective and support and/or training services to fulfill that objective.	$ 949 million[d]
Disabled Veterans Outreach Program (DVOP)	DVOP funds state personnel positions that provide intensive employment services to disabled and other high-need veterans.	$165 million appropriation from DOL (also funds LVER)

Program	Description	FY2012 Funding
Specialized versions of other programs	TAP, Federal hiring preference, and WOTC all have specialized components that target veterans with service-connected disabilities.	Included in general program costs
Competitive Grant Programs that Provide Supplemental Services		
Veterans Workforce Investment Program	VWIP provides competitive grants to public and nonprofit organizations to provide training and/or employment services to veterans.	$14.6 million appropriation from DOL
Collaborative Veterans' Training, Mentoring, and Placement Program	This program provides funds to nonprofit agencies to provide employment-related services to veterans.	$4.5 million appropriation from the VA for two-year program
Veterans Upward Bound (VUB)	VUB provides services such as tutoring and application assistance to aid veterans in preparing for a program of postsecondary education	$13 million appropriation from the Department of Education (ED)

Source: Sources are listed in each program's section of this report.

a. DOD has estimated that its FY2013 costs will increase to $200 million due to the implementation of Transition GPS.

b. Program is an entitlement not subject to appropriations. FY2012 costs are estimates for Post-9/11 GI Bill and Montgomery GI Bill-Active Duty only and do not include administrative expenses.

c. Estimated expenditures for FY2012. The program did not begin until July 1, 2012, so the estimate in the table reflects partial-year expenditures. Estimated expenditures for FY2013, when the program will run the entire fiscal year, are $1.1 billion.

d. Program is an entitlement and not subject to appropriation. FY2012 costs are estimates and include benefits and subsistence allowances; they do not include administrative and counseling expenses.

e. Veteran small business loan programs share funding with non-veteran programs and an estimate limited to veterans' loans is not available. SBA's Office of Veterans Business Development (OVBD) received an appropriation of $2.5 million in FY2012, though SBA used its transfer authority to direct up to $9.3 million to OVBD.

General Veterans' Employment and Training Programs

The programs discussed in this section are available to most veterans of active duty. In the interest of simplicity, this report generally does not present detailed eligibility criteria for each program and benefit, though it does attempt to note eligibility requirements that categorically exclude large numbers of veterans (such as the eligibility window following discharge for GI Bill benefits). This report may omit requirements that would exclude relatively few veterans, such as most programs' exclusion of veterans who were dishonorably discharged.[12] The specific eligibility criteria for each program will usually be available in the external sources that are referenced in the report section that discusses the program.

Transition Programs for Separating Members of the Armed Forces[13]

In 1990, as the post-Cold War drawdown was beginning, Congress authorized a set of benefits and services to assist military personnel in the transition to civilian life.[14] Some of these authorities continued in effect after the drawdown was complete and formed the basis of the Transition Assistance Program (TAP). TAP is currently undergoing substantial modification. A pilot program, Transition Goals Plans Success (Transition GPS), is underway and is expected to completely replace TAP by the end of 2013.[15] Both programs are described below.

Transition Assistance Program (TAP)

TAP provides pre-separation services and counseling on a number of transition-related topics to separating members of the Armed Forces. In addition to guidance on broader transition issues such as financial management and health care, TAP includes information on the following employment issues as they relate to veterans:

- the correlation between military skills and civilian occupations;
- professional certifications, including licensing and apprenticeships;
- public and community service opportunities, including federal employment opportunities and veterans' hiring preferences (described in a subsequent section of this report);
- self-employment and entrepreneurship, including veterans' small business and entrepreneurship programs; and
- education and training assistance, including use of veterans' educational benefits and other job training opportunities.

Separating personnel can also elect to participate in a three-day employment workshop, which covers skills such as choosing a career, conducting job searches, interviewing, and writing cover letters and resumes, as well as providing analyses of employment conditions in various occupations and the labor market at large. Separating personnel can also opt to attend a four hour veterans' benefits brief sponsored by the VA.

A Disabled Transition Assistance Program (DTAP) also exists within TAP. In addition to the above mentioned services, DTAP includes individual instruction for disabled service members regarding their job-readiness and special needs they might have as a result of their disability, along with information on the VA's Vocational Rehabilitation and Employment services (described later in this report).

TAP services are provided at many military installations, often found in the military installation's career or family support offices. The Department of Defense (DOD), Department of Labor (DOL), Department of Veterans Affairs (VA), and the Department of Homeland Security (DHS) are each involved in conducting TAP.[16]

Transition GPS

Transition GPS is the name of the redesigned transition assistance program brought about by the work of the executive branch's Veterans' Employment Initiative Task Force and intended to conform with the Veterans Opportunity to Work (VOW) to Hire Heroes Act of 2011.[17] Among other changes, the VOW Act made participation in TAP mandatory for nearly all separating military personnel and required that each TAP participant receive "an individualized assessment of the various positions of civilian employment in the private sector for which such member may be qualified" as a result of their military training. These statutory changes took effect on November 21, 2012, one year after the enactment of the VOW Act.

DOD introduced the Transition GPS pilot program at seven military bases in the summer of 2012. It includes a five-day core program that incorporates the elements of TAP described above into a redesigned curriculum. Some of the key differences between TAP and Transition GPS include

- the five-day core curriculum is mandatory, not optional, for nearly all separating servicemembers;
- class sizes will be smaller to provide individual attention;
- the individual transition plan is standardized, tied to the servicemembers personal goals, and includes a "skills-gap" analysis;
- successful completion is based on achieving "career readiness standards," not simply attendance;
- the program concludes with a "capstone event" to verify that career readiness standards have been achieved; and

- in addition to the core curriculum, servicemembers will be able to participate in optional tracks for education, entrepreneurship, and technical training.

The "core" Transition GPS curriculum was implemented in November 2012. The optional tracks are expected to be implemented by the end of 2013.

GI Bill Educational Assistance Programs[18]

The VA administers several educational assistance programs for veterans (commonly known as GI Bills) that are intended to avert unemployment, adjust veterans to civilian life, reward military service, encourage recruitment and retention in the military, and make education affordable. VA educational assistance payments are available for approved programs of education as well as living expenses while enrolled.[19]

While there are several GI Bill programs, the vast majority of veterans who utilize education benefits do so under the Post-9/11 GI Bill or the Montgomery GI Bill-Active Duty (MGIB-AD). Both programs provide benefits for 36 months of full-time schooling or the equivalent in part- time attendance.[20] The Post-9/11 GI Bill provides separate payments for tuition and fees, supplies, housing, and other costs. The maximum benefit for tuition and fees at a public institution of higher learning is equal to in-state tuition and fees for that program of education. As of August 1, 2012, the maximum benefit for tuition and fees at a private or foreign institution is $18,078 per academic year. The monthly housing allowance under the Post-9/11 GI Bill varies by geographical location and ranges from $765 in the Mansfield, Ohio area to $2,835 in the New York City area.[21] MGIB-AD provides a single monthly payment to the veteran to cover both education and living expenses. As of October 1, 2012, the maximum benefit under MGIB-AD is $1,564 per month.

Post 9/11 GI Bill benefits are typically available within 15 years of discharge or release from active duty. MGIB-AD benefits (and most other GI Bill benefits) are generally available within ten years. Notably, GI Bill benefits are not considered when calculating a student's eligibility for need-based Pell grants, meaning that a veteran who meets Pell grant criteria may receive both Pell grants and GI Bill benefits.[22] As an additional benefit, educational assistance received under a VA education program (including subsistence or housing allowances for enrolled veterans) is not subject to federal income tax.

In its FY2013 budget, the VA estimated that in total FY2012 benefits for the Post-9/11 GI Bill and Montgomery GI Bill-Active Duty were $10.5 billion.[23]

Veterans Retraining Assistance Program (VRAP)[24]

The VRAP program was created by the VOW Act to provide employment-related training for older unemployed veterans who were no longer eligible for the GI Bill.[25] It provides up to 12 months of training benefits to unemployed veterans who are not eligible for other VA education programs and are between the ages of 35 and 60.[26] It is administered by the VA.

VRAP benefits are limited to training at community colleges or technical schools in occupations that DOL has identified as "high demand."[27] Monthly benefit levels are limited to the maximum amounts under the MGIB-AD program (described in the previous section). While benefits are limited to 12 months, veterans may enroll in programs longer than 12 months. In cases where a program is less than 12 months, benefits are limited to the duration of the program.

VRAP is limited to 45,000 participants from July 1, 2012 to September 30, 2012 and 54,000 participants from October 1, 2012 to March 31, 2014. The VA has estimated that in FY2013, the first full year of the program, VRAP obligations will be $1.1 billion.[28]

Local Veterans Employment Representatives (LVER) Employment Services[29]

The LVER program provides formula grants to states to hire personnel that provide assistance to veterans who are seeking employment.[30] LVER staff provide employment services to veterans and conduct outreach to local employers to develop employment opportunities for veterans. Outreach activities might include advocacy efforts to local employers and workshops for veterans seeking employment. LVER staff are familiar with a range of veteran services and may provide referral to other entities in the support of veterans seeking employment.

Statute specifies that, "to the maximum extent possible," states should hire veterans as LVER personnel, with the highest preference is given to veterans with service-connected disabilities who are otherwise qualified for the position.[31] LVER personnel work in conjunction with the One-Stop delivery system, and are often physically stationed at One-Stop Career Centers, as established by the Workforce Investment Act of 1998 (WIA; P.L. 105-220).[32]

The LVER program is part of the Jobs for Veterans State Grant (JVSG) program, which is administered by the Veterans Employment and Training Service (VETS) of DOL.[33] JVSG also provides funds for the Disabled Veterans Outreach Program (DVOP), which is described in a subsequent section of this report. In FY2012, JVSG's budget authority was approximately $165 million. JVSG is funded out of the Employment Security Administration Account in the Unemployment Trust Fund.

Priority of Service in DOL-Funded Training and Employment Service Programs

In addition to veteran-targeted programs, DOL administers a number of public programs to assist individuals in training for and securing employment. These services include subsidized training as well as employment services such as job search assistance and resume preparation. The Jobs for Veterans Act of 2002 (P.L. 107-288) specifies that veterans will receive priority of service in all DOL-funded training programs.[34] DOL has clarified that this includes all services provided at One-Stop Career Centers (including employment services such as job search assistance).[35]

In 2011, DOL launched a Gold Card initiative directed at Post-9/11 veterans. In addition to priority in all training programs, the initiative also provides veterans with intensive employment services such as job readiness assessments, career guidance, and referral to training through WIA, an apprenticeship, or other federal or state programs. Veterans may also receive six months of follow-up services from a case manager.[36]

Skills and Experience Transfer

While there are no appropriated programs that exclusively support the transfer of military skills to the civilian labor market, there are several tools that can assist veterans and service providers (such as TAP administrators and LVER personnel) in identifying occupations that utilize military skills and experience. Examples of these tools include the VA's Military Skills Translator[37] and O*Net's MyNextMove for Veterans[38] (funded by DOL). The National Resource Directory, a veterans-directed collaboration between the Department of Defense (DOD), DOL, and the VA, also has a skills translator that is connected to localized employment listings.[39]

The VOW Act addresses the issue of transferring military skills with a demonstration project that requires DOL to select five military occupational specialties with skills that are transferrable to high-growth civilian industries. DOL then must work with a coalition of federal, state, and private entities to determine what military skills, training, and experience may align with requirements for civilian credentials, certifications, and licenses.[40]

Another law enacted in the 112th Congress related to transferring military experience into civilian credentials. In July 2012, the president signed the Veteran Skills to Jobs Act (P.L. 112-147). The law states that "The Head of each Federal licensing authority shall consider and may accept, in the case of any individual applying for a license, any relevant training received by such individual while serving as a member of the armed forces[.]"

Veterans may also be able to convert their military training, skills, and experience into postsecondary education credit if they enroll in a school that participates in the Servicemembers Opportunity College (SOC) consortium.[41] Institutions in the SOC Consortium agree to adhere to a set of servicemember-focused policies. Among these is the consideration of converting military experience and training into postsecondary credit.

Work Opportunity Tax Credit (WOTC) for Employers[42]

The WOTC provides a tax credit for employers who hire qualified veterans. In cases where the eligible hire works at least 400 hours, the credit is equal to 40% of the wages paid to the eligible veteran, up to a certain level.[43] The VOW Act established the current credit amounts and veteran criteria:[44]

- a maximum credit of $2,400 for hiring a veteran who is receiving Supplemental Nutrition Assistance Program (SNAP; formerly food stamps) benefits for at least three months during the year prior to hire;
- a maximum credit of $2,400 for hiring a veteran who has been unemployed for a total of at least four weeks but less than six months in the year prior to hire;
- a maximum credit of $4,800 for hiring a veteran who is eligible for disability compensation from the VA and is within one year of discharge or release from military duty;
- a maximum credit of $5,600 for hiring a veteran who has been unemployed for a total of at least six months in the year prior to hire; and
- a maximum credit of $9,600 for hiring a veteran who is eligible for disability compensation from the VA and who has been unemployed for a total of six months in the year prior to hire.

In addition to veterans, the WOTC is also available to employers that employ individuals in other target populations (e.g., at-risk youth or convicted felons). The WOTC for both veteran and nonveteran groups is set to expire on December 31, 2013.

Federal Employment[45]

There are several programs and policies that provide a preference for veterans in obtaining employment in the federal government. These policies and programs can either give veterans an advantage in the competitive hiring process or, in some cases, allow a veteran to be appointed without going through the competitive process.

Points Preference

In the federal hiring process for competitive positions, candidates may be evaluated through a system that assigns point values to relevant experience, skills, and education. Depending on the specifics of their active military service, veterans may receive extra points added to their numerical score.

A five-point preference is available to veterans who served after September 11, 2001.[46] A five point-preference is also available to veterans who served during specified wartimes or in specified campaigns.[47] A ten-point preference is available to veterans who either (1) have a service-connected disability or (2) received a Purple Heart. The ten-point preference is available to these veterans regardless of their period or location of service.

Special Hiring Authorities

There are several hiring programs that allow qualified veterans to be appointed to what would otherwise be competitive federal positions without having to compete with the general public. Typically, these programs allow an agency to hire a veteran in a shorter period of time than it would take to fill the position through the competitive service process. To be eligible for these special hiring authorities, a veteran must be have been separated from the Armed Forces for less than three years, have served in a qualified combat mission, or be disabled.[48]

Other Initiatives

In 2009, President Barack Obama issued Executive Order 13518, which aimed to "enhance recruitment of and promote employment opportunities for veterans within the executive branch[.]"[49] The program established a Council on Veterans Employment that included 24 agencies and required each agency to develop an agency-specific plan and designate an office or officer for promoting employment opportunities for veterans within the agency. The order also established a website that offered veteran-specific information on obtaining federal employment as well as contact information for the individual or office in each agency responsible for promoting veterans' employment within the agency.[50]

The VOW Act expanded on this effort by directing the Office of Personnel Management (OPM) to (1) designate agencies to establish a program to provide employment assistance to separating service members and (2) ensure that those programs are coordinated with the Transition Assistance Program for existing service members (discussed later in this report).

Small Business Administration Programs

The Small Business Administration (SBA) has a variety of programs to assist veterans with developing and managing a small business, financing a small business, and acquiring federal contracts.[51] Congressional interest in these programs has increased in recent years primarily due to reports by veteran organizations that veterans were experiencing difficulty accessing the SBA's programs, especially the Patriot Express Pilot Loan Guaranty Program, as well as general interest in facilitating the transition of veterans from military to civilian life.

The SBA currently provides management and technical assistance training services to veterans through its various management and technical assistance training partners and responds to veteran inquires through its SBA district offices.[52] The SBA's Patriot Express Pilot Loan Guaranty Program is a component of SBA's larger 7(a) lending program, available only to veterans, certain active military service people, and certain spouses.[53] The loan proceeds can be used for expansion, renovation, new construction, the purchase of land or buildings, the purchase of equipment, working capital, etc. The Patriot Express program differs from the general 7(a) program in that it features streamlined documentation and processing features, has a lower loan limit (up to $500,000), and has a targeted SBA processing time of one business day.

The SBA also assists small businesses, including service-disabled veteran-owned small businesses, in acquiring federal contracts through its management and oversight of the federal government's procurement goals for small businesses.[54] Under the Small Business Goaling program, at least 3% of the total value of all small business eligible prime contract awards and subcontract awards are supposed to be awarded to small businesses owned and controlled by service-disabled veteran-owned small businesses.[55]

Programs for Veterans with Service-Connected Disabilities

Dedicated employment services exist for veterans with service-connected disabilities. The Vocational Rehabilitation and Employment (VR&E) program provides comprehensive services for veterans with a service-connected disability and does not have an analogue among general veterans' program. Other programs for disabled veterans are specialized variations of general programs that were discussed previously.

Vocational Rehabilitation and Employment (VR&E)[56]

VR&E provides job training and employment services to veterans who have service-connected disabilities.[57] To be entitled to VR&E services, a veteran with a service-connected disability must also demonstrate an employment handicap that hinders the veteran's ability to prepare for, obtain, or retain employment consistent with his or her abilities, aptitudes, and interests.

VR&E offers several tracks of services, depending on the veteran's employment objective and needs. Veterans who already have the necessary job skills or seek to return to previous employment can receive short-term services such as resume assistance and job accommodations. Veterans who need job skills are eligible for education and training benefits as well as employment services once they complete training. The VA has reported that long-term services, including training, is the most-utilized VR&E track.

In FY2012, VR&E benefits are estimated to be approximately $949 million. Program administration, including counseling, are estimated to be an additional $204 million.[58]

Disabled Veterans Outreach Program (DVOP) Employment Services[59]

DVOP provides formula grants to states to hire staff to provide a range of intensive services to veterans with service-connected disabilities as well as other veterans with multiple barriers to employment.[60] Services include case management, referral to other service providers (e.g., the VA's VR&E program discussed in the prior subsection), employment counseling, and job search assistance.

DVOP is part of DOL's JVSG program, which also funds the previously discussed LVER program.[61] In FY2012, JVSG's budget authority was approximately $165 million. JVSG is funded out of the Employment Security Administration Account in the Unemployment Trust Fund.

Components of General Programs that Target Disabled Veterans

Several of the broader veterans programs described previously in this report, have specialized components for disabled veterans. Additional detail can be found in the sources referenced in each program's primary section of this report.

- *Transition Assistance Program.* The Disabled Transition Assistance Program (DTAP), provides specialized services for exiting service members with service- connected disabilities.
- *Federal Employment.* As discussed in the section above, veterans with a service- connected disability are eligible for the highest preference in competitively-hired federal positions. Disabled veterans are also eligible for special hiring authorities, including noncompetitive appointments for qualified veterans with a disability rating of 30% or more from the VA.[62]
- *Work Opportunity Tax Credit.* Some WOTCs are available for businesses that hire veterans who are eligible for disability compensation from the VA. The largest available tax credit is for hiring a veteran who is eligible for disability compensation and who was unemployed for at least 6 of the 12 months prior to hire.

Veteran-Targeted Competitive Grant Programs

Additional programs provide competitive grants for entities that provide services to veterans. Since the programs are competitive grants, they may only be available in certain areas, may have limited capacity, or may only serve a targeted veteran population.

The programs discussed below do not include competitive grant programs that include employment services as part of a broader group of services. For example, the employment components of the Homeless Veterans Reintegration Program are omitted.[63]

TRIO Veterans Upward Bound (VUB)[64]

The TRIO Veterans Upward Bound (VUB) program provides services to assist veterans in preparing for a program of postsecondary education. VUB projects provide academic instruction, tutoring, assistance in completing secondary school, assistance with college admissions and applications, and assistance applying for financial assistance. It is administered by the Department of Education (ED).

To be eligible for participation, veterans must be in need of academic support to pursue education beyond secondary school successfully. At least two-thirds of program participants must be low- income, potential first-generation college students. The remaining one-third of participants must be either low-income, potential first generation college students, or otherwise be at-risk of academic failure. The program defines a veteran who is at-risk for academic failure as an individual who has been out of high school or dropped out of a program of postsecondary education for five or more years; has scored on standardized tests below the level that demonstrates a likelihood of success in a program of postsecondary education; or meets the definition of an individual with a disability.

In 2012, ED allocated $14 million of the $840 million FY2012 TRIO appropriation to VUB projects.[65]

Veterans Workforce Investment Program (VWIP)[66]

WIA authorizes grants for programs to meet the needs of "veterans with service-connected disabilities, veterans who have significant barriers to employment, veterans who served on active duty in the Armed Forces during a war or in a campaign or expedition for which a campaign badge has been authorized, and recently separated veterans." Programs may contain training or other employment services.

In FY2012, $14.6 million was appropriated for these grants. A 2012 Solicitation for Grant Applications expressed an intention of awarding grants ranging from $750,000 to $1,250,000 for a three-year period of performance.[67]

Collaborative Veterans' Training, Mentoring, and Placement Program

The VOW Act requires the VA to award grants to nonprofit agencies to "to provide training and mentoring for eligible veterans who seek employment." Grant recipients are required to collaborate with local DVOP personnel as well as state and local workforce agencies to "facilitate the placement of the veterans that complete the training in meaningful employment that leads to economic self-sufficiency."[68]

This program is smaller than the other competitive grant programs discussed in this section. The VOW Act authorizes a total of $4.5 million to carry out this activity in FY2012 and FY2013. The VOW Act specifies that grants will go to no more than three organizations.

End Notes

[1] References also include a CRS analyst to contact about the topic. In cases where a topic does not list a contact, inquiries should be directed to the coordinator of this report.

[2] This section was prepared by Benjamin Collins, Analyst in Labor Policy, bcollins@crs.loc.gov, 7-7382.

[3] The designation of Gulf War II veterans follows the definition set by the Bureau of Labor Statistics. Data for veterans from other periods were calculated by subtracting Gulf War II veterans data from total veterans data.

[4] In **Table 1** and **Figure 1**, CRS calculated quarterly estimates by aggregating monthly data to control for large month- to-month fluctuations.

[5] Data on veterans' characteristics are 2011 annual averages and from Bureau of Labor Statistics, "Employment Situation of Veterans—2011," March 20, 2012, http://www.bls.gov/news.release/vet.htm. Monthly data on veterans' characteristics are not published by BLS. Data for 2012 will be released in March 2013.

[6] Ibid. Table 2A.

[7] Ibid. Table 3. Data only consider veterans age 25 and over. About 11% of the GWII veterans in the labor force are under the age of 25.

[8] Ibid. Table 6. Approximately 17% of veterans did not report their disability status and were excluded from this analysis.

[9] The reference period was determined by the earliest availability of monthly data for GWII veterans.

[10] While aggregating monthly data into quarterly totals somewhat reduces the dynamism of these estimates, the unemployment rate for GWII veterans still fluctuates more than larger populations.

[11] 2005 was the first year that BLS published data on GWII veterans. Data are available from "The Employment Situation of Veterans" press releases from BLS, archived at http://www.bls.gov/schedule/archives/all_nr.htm#VET. "The Employment Situation of Veterans" has been an annual release since 2007. Prior to 2007, it was issued on a biennial basis.

[12] For a more detailed discussion factors that may influence a former service member's eligibility for veterans' benefits, see CRS Report R42324, *"Who is a Veteran?"—Basic Eligibility for Veterans' Benefits*, by Christine Scott.

[13] This section written by Lawrence Kapp, Specialist in Military Manpower Policy (x7-7609) and Fenwick Gilroy, Research Associate.

[14] Codified at 10 U.S.C. 1141-1150.

[15] Terri Cronk, "New Program Aims to Better Help Troops Transition to Civilian Life," American Forces Press Service, August 18, 2012, available at http://www.detnese.gov/news/newsarticle.aspx?id=117544.

[16] Memorandum of Understanding between the Department of Labor, Department of Defense, Department of Veterans Affairs, and Department of Homeland Security, "Transition Assistance Program and Disabled Transition Assistance Program," signed September 19, 2006, available at http://www.dol.gov/vets/vpls/VPL%20Attachments/VPL%201-08%20Attch%201%20-%20Transition%20Assistance%20and%20Disabled%20Transition%20Assistance%20Programs%20Memorandum%20of%20Understanding%20dated%20September%2019,%202007.pdf.

[17] The VOW to Hire Heroes Act is Title II of P.L. 112-56. In addition to modifying TAP, the law had other provisions related to veterans' employment. The VOW to Hire Heroes Act will be referred to as "the VOW Act" throughout this report.

[18] For more information on each of the GI Bills, see CRS Report R42785, *GI Bills Enacted Prior to 2008 and Related Veterans' Educational Assistance Programs: A Primer*, by Cassandria Dortch, and CRS Report R42755, *The Post-9/11 Veterans Educational Assistance Act of 2008 (Post-9/11 GI Bill): Primer and Issues*, by Cassandria Dortch.

[19] Eligible educational programs include but are not limited to college courses, vocational programs, entrepreneurship courses, apprenticeships, on-the-job training, and licensing or certification tests.

[20] Benefits can be used in nonconsecutive months. For example, a veteran may use GI Bill benefits for four traditional nine-month full-time academic years.

[21] Monthly housing allowances under the Post-9/11 GI Bill equal the monthly basic allowance for housing for a member of the Armed Forces with dependents in pay grade E-5 in the military housing area in which the veteran's educational institution is located. Local rates are available at http://www.defensetravel.dod.mil/Docs/perdiem/browse/ Allowances/BAH/ PDF/2012/2012-With-Dependents-BAH-Rates.pdf.

[22] For more information on Pell Grants, see CRS Report R42446, *Federal Pell Grant Program of the Higher Education Act: How the Program Works, Recent Legislative Changes, and Current Issues*, by Shannon M. Mahan.

[23] The FY2013 budget was issued in February 2012. See Volume III of the FY2013 VA Budget, page 2B-2 at http://www.va.gov/budget/docs/summary/Fy2013_Volume_III-Benefits_ Burial_Dept_Admin.pdf.

[24] For more information on the VRAP program, including current application procedures and current enrollment levels, see http://benefits.va.gov/vow/education.htm.

[25] VRAP was created by Section 211 of P.L. 112-56.

[26] Veterans are ineligible for VRAP if they received a dishonorable discharge, are receiving VA compensation due to unemployability, or are enrolled in a federal or state job training program.

[27] The VA has identified more than 200 occupations as eligible for VRAP benefits. See http://benefits.va.gov/vow/ docs/VRAP_High_Demand.pdf for the complete list.

[28] See Volume III of the FY2013 VA Budget, page 2B-2 at http://www.va.gov/budget/docs/ summary/Fy2013_Volume_III-Benefits_Burial_Dept_ Admin.pdf.

[29] This section was prepared by David H. Bradley, Specialist in Labor Economics, dbradley@crs.loc.gov, 7-7352.

[30] LVER is codified at 38 U.S.C. 4104.

[31] See 38 U.S.C. 4104(c).

[32] For more information on WIA and One-Stop Career Centers, see CRS Report R41135, *The Workforce Investment Act and the One-Stop Delivery System*, by David H. Bradley.

[33] More information on veteran-related initiatives administered the U.S. Department of Labor, including the JVSG program, is available at http://www.dol.gov/vets/.

[34] To receive priority of service, a veteran must meet the program's eligibility criteria regarding age, employment history, or other characteristics.

[35] See 20 C.F.R. 1010.200-330.

[36] More information on the Gold Card initiative is available at http://www.dol.gov/vets/ goldcard.html.

[37] See https://mst.vaforvets.va.gov/mst/va/mos-translator.

[38] See http://www.mynextmove.org/vets/.

[39] See https://www.nrd.gov/home/veterans_job_bank.

[40] See P.L. 112-56, Section 237 and 38 U.S.C. 4114.

[41] The SOC consortium is privately administered. For more information on the Consortium, see http://www.soc.aascu.org/.

[42] For more information on the WOTC, see CRS Report RL30089, *The Work Opportunity Tax Credit (WOTC)*, by Christine Scott. This report also describes nonveteran populations that are eligible for the WOTC.

[43] The size of the WOTC is based on wages paid the employee during the first year of employment. In cases where an eligible hire works between 120 and 400 hours, the tax credit is reduced to 25% of wages paid. If the eligible hire works fewer than 120 hours, the employer is not eligible for the credit.

[44] Under the VOW Act, the WOTC was limited to veterans and set to expire on December 31, 2012. Section 309 of P.L. 112-240 reinstated the WOTC for all populations through December 31, 2013.

[45] For a more in-depth discussion of federal employment for veterans, see CRS Report RS22666, *Veterans Benefits: Federal Employment Assistance*, by Christine Scott.

[46] The service period under this criteria is set to end on the date prescribed by Presidential proclamation or law as the last date of Operation Iraqi Freedom. As of this writing, no such proclamation or law has been issued.

[47] Applicable dates and criteria are available from the Office of Personnel Management at http://www.opm.gov/ staffingportal/vetguide.asp#2When.

[48] Full details on these hiring authorities is available from the Office of Personnel Management at http://www.opm.gov/ staffingportal/vetguide.asp#6.

[49] The full text of the order, including a list of participating agencies, is available at http://www.gpo.gov/fdsys/pkg/FR- 2009-11-13/pdf/E9-27441.pdf.

[50] See http://www.fedshirevets.gov/AgencyDirectory/index.aspx for a list of agency contacts.

[51] See CRS Report R42695, *SBA Veterans Assistance Programs: An Analysis of Contemporary Issues*, by Robert Jay Dilger and Sean Lowry.

[52] See CRS Report R41352, *Small Business Management and Technical Assistance Training Programs*, by Robert Jay Dilger.

[53] See CRS Report R41146, *Small Business Administration 7(a) Loan Guaranty Program*, by Robert Jay Dilger, and U.S. Small Business Administration, "SOP 50 10 5(E): Lender and Development Company Loan Programs," (effective June 1, 2012), pp. 83, 127, at http://www.sba.gov/sites/default/files/SOP%2050%2010%205(E)%20(5-16-012)%20clean.pdf.

[54] See CRS Report RL33243, *Small Business Administration: A Primer on Programs*, by Robert Jay Dilger and Sean Lowry.

[55] See P.L. 100-656, the Business Opportunity Development Reform Act of 1988 and P.L. 105-135, the HUBZone Act of 1997 —Title VI of the Small Business Reauthorization Act of 1997 (small businesses generally); and P.L. 106-50, the Veterans Entrepreneurship and Small Business Development Act of 1999 (service-disabled veteran owned).

[56] For more information on the VR&E program, see CRS Report RL34627, *Veterans' Benefits: The Vocational Rehabilitation and Employment Program*, by Benjamin Collins.

[57] VR&E also provides independent living services to veterans who are not able to work. In FY2011, approximately 25% of completed rehabilitations under VR&E were independent living (i.e., not employment-based) rehabilitations.

[58] See Volume III of the FY2012 VA budget at http://www.va.gov/budget/docs/summary/ Fy2013_Volume_III-Benefits_Burial_ Dept_Admin.pdf.

[59] This section was prepared by David H. Bradley, Specialist in Labor Economics, dbradley@crs.loc.gov, 7-7352.

[60] DVOP is codified at 38 U.S.C. 4103A.

[61] JVSG is described in greater detail in the "Local Veterans Employment Representatives (LVER) Employment Services" section of this report. More information on veteran-related initiatives administered the U.S. Department of Labor, including the JVSG program, is available at http://www.dol.gov/vets/.

[62] For more information on the "30% or More Disabled Veterans" hiring authority, see http://www.opm.gov/ staffingportal/vetguide.asp#30%Disabled.

[63] The Homeless Veterans Reintegration Program is discussed in CRS Report RL34024, *Veterans and Homelessness*, by Libby Perl.

[64] For more information on TRIO programs, including Upward Bound, see CRS Report R42724, *The TRIO Programs: A Primer*, by Cassandria Dortch.

[65] U.S. Department of Education, Veterans Upward Bound Program, Funding Status, http://www2.ed.gov/programs/ triovub/funding.html, as downloaded on January 4, 2013.

[66] VWIP is authorized by Section 168 of WIA. Questions on VWIP should be directed to David H. Bradley, dbradley@crs.loc.gov, 7-7352.

[67] See for more information on VWIP, including the PY2012 SGA, see http://www.dol.gov/vets/ programs/vwip/ main.htm.

[68] See Section 234 of P.L. 112-56.

In: Veterans
Editor: Timothy C. Roberts
ISBN: 978-1-63117-046-1

Chapter 4

VA VOCATIONAL REHABILITATION AND EMPLOYMENT PROGRAM: IMPROVED OVERSIGHT OF INDEPENDENT LIVING SERVICES AND SUPPORTS IS NEEDED*

United States Government Accountability Office

WHY GAO DID THIS STUDY

The IL "track"—one of five tracks within VA's VR&E program—provides a range of benefits to help veterans with service-connected disabilities live independently when employment is not considered feasible at the time they enter the VR&E program. These benefits can include counseling, assistive devices, and other services or equipment. GAO was asked to review issues related to the IL track. This report examines (1) the characteristics of veterans in the IL track, and the types and costs of benefits they were provided; (2) the extent to which their IL plans were completed, and the time it took to complete them; and (3) the extent to which the IL track has been administered appropriately and consistently across regional offices.

* This is an edited, reformatted and augmented version of the Highlights of GAO-13-474, a report to congressional requesters, dated June, 2013.

To conduct this work, GAO analyzed VA administrative data from fiscal years 2008 to 2011, and reviewed a random, generalizable sample of 182 veterans who entered the IL track in fiscal year 2008. In addition, GAO visited five VA regional offices; interviewed agency officials and staff; and reviewed relevant federal laws, regulations, and agency policies and procedures.

WHAT GAO RECOMMENDS

GAO recommends that VR&E explore options to enhance coordination with VHA; strengthen its oversight of the IL track; and reassess its policy for approving benefits. VA generally agreed with GAO's conclusions and recommendations.

WHAT GAO FOUND

Of the 9,215 veterans who entered the Department of Veterans Affairs' (VA) Independent Living (IL) track within the Vocational Rehabilitation and Employment (VR&E) program in fiscal years 2008 to 2011, most were male Vietnam era veterans in their 50s or 60s. Almost 60 percent served in the U.S. Army, and fewer than 1 percent served in the National Guard or Reserve. The most prevalent disabilities among these veterans were post-traumatic stress disorder and tinnitus. GAO's review of 182 IL cases from fiscal year 2008 found that VR&E provided a range of IL benefits to veterans. Among these cases, the most common benefits were counseling services and computers. Less common benefits included gym memberships, camping equipment, and a boat. GAO estimated that VR&E spent nearly $14 million on benefits for veterans entering the IL track in fiscal year 2008—an average of almost $6,000 per IL veteran.

Most veterans completed their IL plans, which identify their individual goals to live independently and the benefits VR&E will provide. About 89 percent of fiscal year 2008 IL veterans were considered by VR&E to be "rehabilitated," that is, generally, to have completed their IL plans by the end of fiscal year 2011. VR&E discontinued or closed about 5 percent of cases for various reasons, such as the veteran declined benefits. Six percent of cases were open at the end of fiscal year 2011. Because the complexity of IL cases varied depending on veterans' disabilities and needs, some cases were fairly simple for VR&E to close. For example, one IL case only called for the installation of door levers and a bathtub rail. Another more complex case involved the provision of a range of IL benefits, including home modifications. Rehabilitation rates across regions varied from 0 to 100 percent, and regions with larger IL caseloads generally rehabilitated a greater percentage of IL veterans. While IL plans nationwide were completed in 384 days, on average, completion times varied by region, from 150 to 895 days.

VR&E exercises limited oversight to ensure appropriate and consistent administration of the IL track across its regions. First, some regions may not be complying with certain case management requirements. For instance, while VR&E is required to coordinate with the Veterans Health Administration (VHA) on IL benefits, VR&E counselors have difficulty obtaining timely responses from VHA. VHA physicians respond to VR&E's IL referrals late or not at all, resulting in delayed benefits or VR&E providing the benefits instead of VHA. Second, VR&E does not monitor regional variation in IL caseloads and benefits provided. Instead, it has relied on its quality assurance reviews and ad hoc studies, but these are limited in scope. Third, given counselors have broad discretion in selecting IL benefits, VR&E's written policies for approving IL expenditures may not be appropriate as regions were permitted to purchase a range of items without any Central Office approval, some of which were costly or questionable. For example, in one case, Central Office review would not have been required for expenditures of $18,829 for a riding mower, which is prohibited, and other items. Finally, VR&E's system does not collect IL costs and benefits provided. VR&E also lacks accurate data on the number of IL veterans served. While the law currently allows 2,700 veterans to enter the IL track annually, data used to monitor the cap are based on the number of IL plans developed, not on the number of individual veterans admitted. Veterans can have more than one plan in a fiscal year, so one veteran could be counted multiple times towards the cap.

ABBREVIATIONS

IL	Independent Living
PSAS	Prosthetics and Sensory Aids Service
PTSD	Post-traumatic Stress Disorder
SAH	Specially Adapted Housing
QA	Quality Assurance
VA	Department of Veterans Affairs

VBA	Veterans Benefits Administration
VHA	Veterans Health Administration
VRC	Vocational Rehabilitation Counselor
VR&E	Vocational Rehabilitation and Employment

June 7, 2013

The Honorable Bill Flores
Chairman
The Honorable Mark Takano
Ranking Member
Subcommittee on Economic Opportunity
Committee on Veterans' Affairs
House of Representatives

The Honorable Bruce Braley
House of Representatives

The Honorable Marlin Stutzman
House of Representatives

The Department of Veterans Affairs' (VA) Vocational Rehabilitation and Employment (VR&E) program, under the Veterans Benefits Administration (VBA), administers five "tracks" that provide a wide range of services and assistance to support veterans with service-connected disabilities. Four of VR&E's five tracks are intended to help veterans prepare for, find, and maintain suitable employment. If employment is not considered a feasible goal for veterans when they enter the VR&E program, they can be assigned to the Independent Living (IL) track for separate, non-employment support within the VR&E program, and can receive benefits such as counseling, assistive devices, and other services or equipment to improve their ability to live independently. By law, the number of veterans who can be assigned to the IL track each year is limited. There are currently 56 VA regional offices with responsibility for administering VR&E's IL track,[1] and almost 3,000 veterans nationwide were served in this track during fiscal year 2011.

Given the limited information available on those who participate in VR&E's IL track, you asked us to review issues related to the benefits IL track veterans receive, and their outcomes. This report examines (1) the characteristics of veterans who have participated in the IL track, as well as the types and costs of benefits they were provided; (2) the extent to which their IL plans were completed, and the time it took to complete them; and (3) the extent to which the IL track has been administered appropriately and consistently across regional offices.

To provide information on the number, characteristics, and outcomes of veterans who entered the IL track, as well as how long it took VR&E to complete these cases, we analyzed VA administrative data from fiscal years 2008 through 2011.[2] We also used these data to estimate the difference, if any, in the amount of time it took to complete these cases across regional offices, as well as across groups of veterans with various characteristics. To determine the types of goods and services provided to veterans and the direct cost of these benefits, we reviewed the case files of a random sample of 182 veterans who were assigned to the IL track at some point during fiscal year 2008.

To obtain information about how the IL track has been administered, we visited VA regional offices in San Diego, California; Atlanta, Georgia; Detroit, Michigan; Philadelphia, Pennsylvania; and the District of Columbia.[3] We selected these sites because they are geographically diverse and have had differing levels of IL caseloads and rehabilitation rates. At each of these sites we interviewed officials from VR&E, VA's Specially Adapted Housing (SAH) program, and Prosthetic and Sensory Aids Service (PSAS), as well as representatives from local veteran service organizations. We also interviewed VR&E officials at the national level, and relied on our case file review to determine the extent to which VR&E, SAH, and PSAS coordinate in the provision of goods and services to IL track veterans. Lastly, we reviewed relevant federal laws and regulations, standards for internal controls and managerial cost accounting, as well as VR&E policies, procedures, and other relevant studies and documentation.

We conducted this performance audit from February 2012 to June 2013 in accordance with generally accepted government auditing standards. Those standards require that we plan and perform the audit to obtain sufficient, appropriate evidence to provide a reasonable basis for our findings and conclusions based on our audit objectives. We believe that the evidence obtained provides a reasonable basis for our findings and conclusions based on our audit objectives. Additional information on our scope and methodology is provided in appendices I and II.

VR&E's Five Tracks at a Glance

Employment-Related Tracks

- **Reemployment:** For veterans who need assistance returning to their previous employer.
- **Rapid Access to Employment:** For veterans with existing skills who are looking for immediate employment.
- **Self-Employment:** For veterans who have the skills to start a business, and for whom self-employment is the best or only option for successful rehabilitation.
- **Employment Through Long-Term Services:** For veterans who need specialized training and/or education to obtain employment.

Independent Living Track

- **Independent Living:** For veterans who are unable to work and need services to live more independently at the time they enter the VR&E program.

Background

VR&E's IL Track

VBA's VR&E program is responsible for implementing five tracks that provide a variety of services and assistance to veterans with service- connected disabilities. Four of the five tracks are designed to help veterans prepare for, find, and maintain suitable employment. VR&E's fifth track—the IL track—generally helps veterans maximize their ability to live independently when the achievement of an employment goal is not considered feasible at the time they enter the VR&E program.[4] To assist these veterans, the law allows VR&E broad discretion in determining the types of services that can be provided to address their needs.[5] When assessing each veteran, VR&E focuses not only on assisting veterans with activities of daily living,[6] but also on veteran's emotional needs and avocational and leisure interests, among other areas.[7] Furthermore, unlike VR&E's employment-related tracks, the law caps the number of veterans who can be admitted into the IL track annually. While this number has increased over the years, the cap was 2,600 veterans in fiscal year

2011 and is currently 2,700.[8] VR&E anticipates an increase in future demand for IL benefits.

VR&E's Eligibility Requirements

All veterans are required to meet VR&E's basic entitlement criteria before they are assigned to one of its five tracks. To be entitled to VR&E services, veterans must generally have at least a 20 percent service-connected disability rating and be in need of rehabilitation because of an employment handicap.[9] The period of eligibility for which veterans can receive benefits from VR&E is 12 years and begins on either (1) the date of separation from active military duty, or (2) the date that VA notifies the veteran of his or her service-connected disability rating. The 12-year eligibility period may be deferred or extended if certain conditions prevent the veteran from participating in a rehabilitation program or if a veteran has a serious employment handicap.[10] To be considered for the IL track, veterans must meet all of VR&E's eligibility requirements and be deemed currently unable to pursue an employment goal.[11]

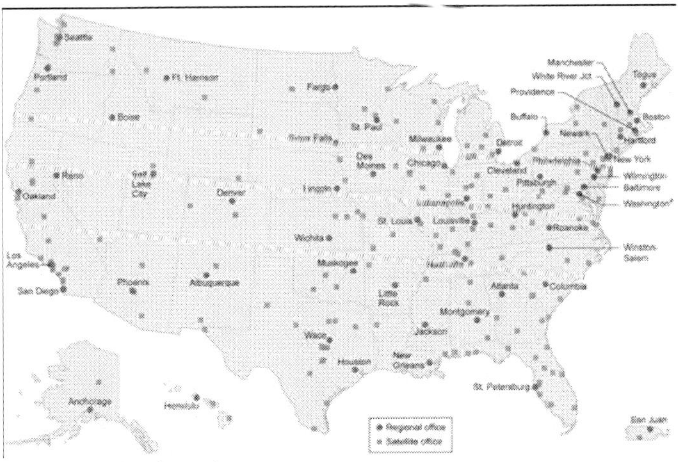

Source: GAO analysis of VA data.

[a] The Washington Regional Office, located in the District of Columbia, was recently designated the National Capital Region Benefits Office in November 2012.

Figure 1. Location of the Vocational Rehabilitation and Employment Program's Regional and Satellite Offices.

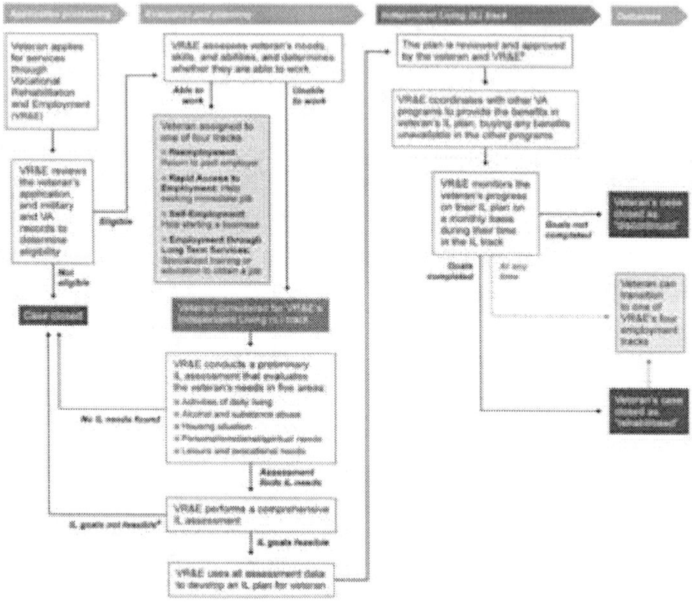

Source: GAO's analysis of VR&E's needs assessment and IL track benefits delivery process.

[a] After both the preliminary and comprehensive IL assessments are performed, a case may be closed if it is determined that the achievement of IL goals are not feasible or if potential needs are not identified. The VR&E officer must concur with this decision.

[b] IL plans must be approved by the VR&E officer, and in some cases the Regional Director or VR&E's Central Office, before any services are provided.

Figure 2. The Vocational Rehabilitation and Employment Program's Needs Assessment and Independent Living Track Benefits Delivery Process.

VR&E's Structure and Administration

VR&E's Central Office, located in Washington D.C., has responsibility for several areas, including (1) overseeing the implementation of the VR&E program, including the IL track, (2) developing program policies and procedures, and regional guidance, and (3) formulating and monitoring the agency's budget and program expenditures. Currently, there are 56 VA regional offices with responsibility for administering the IL track in their jurisdiction.[12] Reporting to these regional offices are 179 satellite offices that help ensure veterans who do not live near a regional office are able to access VR&E benefits, including those provided through the IL track (see figure 1).

The VR&E Officer in each regional office is responsible for ensuring that the office complies with national policies and procedures for monitoring performance to ensure VR&E's national rehabilitation rate is met.[13] In addition, this officer supervises regional Vocational Rehabilitation Counselors (VRCs) who are responsible for working directly with veterans to assess their IL needs and provide benefits.[14]

VR&E has established a formal process that all veterans must go through to receive any of the benefits offered through its five tracks (see figure 2). It is not possible to be assigned to any of the five tracks without first applying and being accepted into the VR&E program.

An individualized IL plan is developed for each veteran admitted to the IL track.[15] This plan identifies the veteran's IL goals, the benefits (goods and services) VR&E will provide to help the veteran meet those goals, estimated time frames for providing benefits, and how improvements in the veteran's independence will be measured, among other areas (see figure 3). In general, IL plans may not exceed 24 months except under certain circumstances.[16] According to officials, there is also no statutory limit on the number of IL plans a veteran can have. Veterans can reapply to the VR&E program at any time.[17]

Furthermore, all IL plans are required to be reviewed and approved by the veteran, the VRC, and the VR&E Officer before the veteran is admitted to the IL track. Once the plan is approved, VRCs are required to meet with the veteran at least once a month to track progress in meeting the plan's goals. In addition, VRCs are required to coordinate with other VA programs to determine if they can provide any of the goods and services identified in the veteran's plan. The VA programs that officials told us they regularly coordinate with are:

- VBA's Specially Adapted Housing (SAH) Program, which helps servicemembers and veterans with certain service-connected disabilities purchase or construct an adapted home, or modify an existing home to accommodate a disability.[18] These modifications can include specially adapted bathrooms or the installation of exit ramps.
- VHA medical centers, which provide a wide range of health-related services to veterans, such as physical therapy and dental and optometry services. In addition, VHA's Prosthetic and Sensory Aids

Service (PSAS) provides a variety of medical devices and equipment to veterans, including artificial limbs, eyeglasses, hearing aids, hospital beds, and wheelchairs.[19] PSAS also administers the Home Improvements and Structural Alterations grant to eligible veterans for home modifications, such as the widening of bedroom or bathroom doorways to allow wheelchair access.

If the goods and services needed cannot be obtained through other VA sources, the VR&E program will purchase them directly or contract for them. VR&E may declare a veteran successfully "rehabilitated" when all goals in their IL plan have been achieved, or if not all achieved, when the following three conditions have been met: (1) the veteran has attained a substantial increase in the level of independence; (2) the veteran has maintained the increased level of independence for at least 60 days; and (3) further assistance is unlikely to significantly increase the veteran's level of independence.[20] "Rehabilitation" does not necessarily mean that a veteran's disability has improved, but rather that the goals in the veteran's IL plan have been met to facilitate their independence. When veterans are not successfully rehabilitated, their case may be closed as "discontinued." When circumstances arise that affect the ability of VR&E to provide the goods and services identified in the IL plan to the veteran, VR&E can temporarily "interrupt" the veteran's case until it becomes possible to continue.

The IL Track Mainly Serves Older Veterans and Provides a Wide Variety of Benefits

IL Serves Mainly Vietnam-Era Veterans and Those with Post-traumatic Stress Disorder

From fiscal years 2008 through 2011, the typical participant in the IL track was an older male Vietnam-era veteran. Of the 9,215 veterans who entered the IL track at some point during these years, most (67 percent) were males 50 years old or older. Most women in the IL track were in their 40s or 50s (see figure 4). The gender and age distributions of IL track veterans were similar to those of veterans who were receiving VA Disability Compensation cash benefits. In fiscal year 2011, about 92 percent of these veterans were male, and almost 68 percent were age 55 or older.

Program goal: Veteran will maximize functional independence in living

	Objective One	*Objective Two*	*Objective Three*	*Objective Four*
	To increase cognitive skills such as memory and concentration through use of cognitive rehabilitation exercises that will be installed on a laptop computer.	Manage stress and anger levels through use of periodic journaling on laptop computer. Veteran will discuss journal activities with social worker, [name], to determine progress for this objective.	Work with a fiduciary for assistance with housing, financial, and organizational issues.	Maintain stability of physical and mental health.
Services provided	Laptop computer with Captain's Log Computerized Cognitive Rehabilitation exercises installed on it and training to use computer.	Laptop computer.	All services necessary to improve ability to manage daily life activities despite the effects of the disability.	Treatment by occupational therapist, social worker, and other medical professionals involved in the well-being of this veteran.
Evaluation criteria	Veteran will develop basic computer skills, and learn how to use Captain's Log. Veteran will attend all scheduled training and practice concepts learned.	Progress will be monitored through self-reports from veteran and reports from treating professionals.	Active participation and cooperation when working with the fiduciary.	Veteran will keep all scheduled medical appointments and follow treatment recommendations, and inform case manager of additional appointment and follow-up referral needs.
Evaluation procedure	Review periodic counseling reports acquired from treating professionals, [name of doctor], verbally or in writing (CAPRI notes).	Review periodic counseling reports acquired from treating professionals verbally or in writing.	Case Manager will monitor veteran's progress through monthly face-to-face visits or by telephone.	Case Manager will monitor veteran's progress in medical and mental health treatment by reviewing medical records and/or speaking with treating professionals.
Evaluation schedule	At least once per month.	At least once per month.	At least once per month.	At least once per month.

Source: GAO analysis of example IL plan provided by VR&E.

Figure 3. Example of an Independent Living Plan Developed for a Veteran.

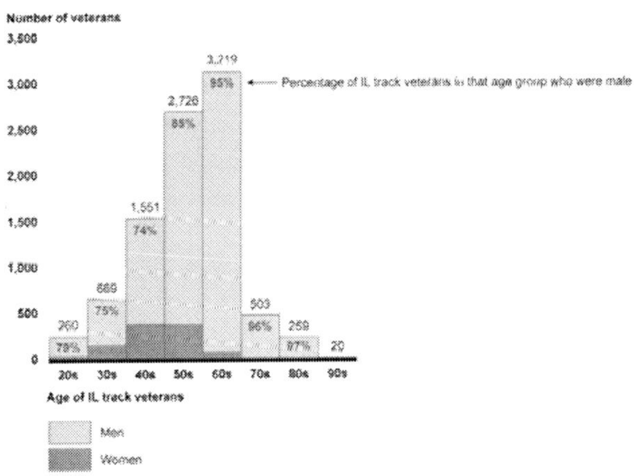

Source: GAO analysis of VA data.

Note: The number in this figure does not add to the 9,215 veterans who entered the IL track during fiscal years 2008 through 2011 because information on gender and age was missing in about 1 percent of these cases.

Figure 4. FY 2008-2011 Independent Living Track Veterans, by Gender and Age.

Most of the 9,215 veterans who entered the IL track during fiscal years 2008 through 2011 served in the Vietnam War. However, there was a slight increase in the number of "Global War on Terrorism" veterans—including those who served during the war in Afghanistan as part of Operation Enduring Freedom and the war in Iraq as part of Operation Iraqi Freedom—from 13 percent in fiscal year 2008 to 16 percent in fiscal year 2011 (see figure 5).

In addition, almost 60 percent of IL track veterans served in the U.S. Army and less than 1 percent served in the National Guard or Reserves. Forty-one percent served in the U.S Navy, U.S. Air Force, or U.S. Marine Corps (see figure 6).

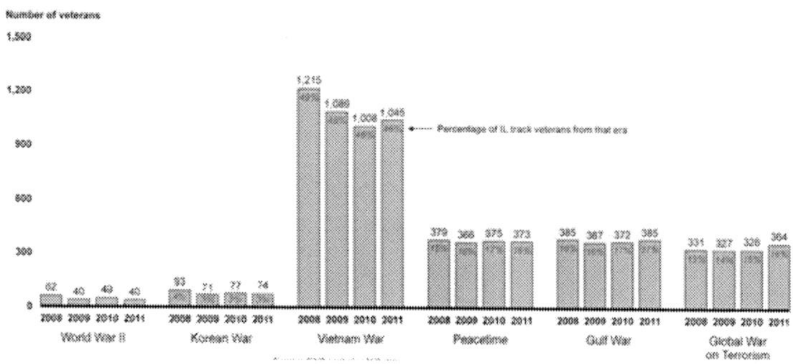

Source: GAO analysis of VA data.

Figure 5. Independent Living Track Veterans during FY 2008-2011, by War Era.

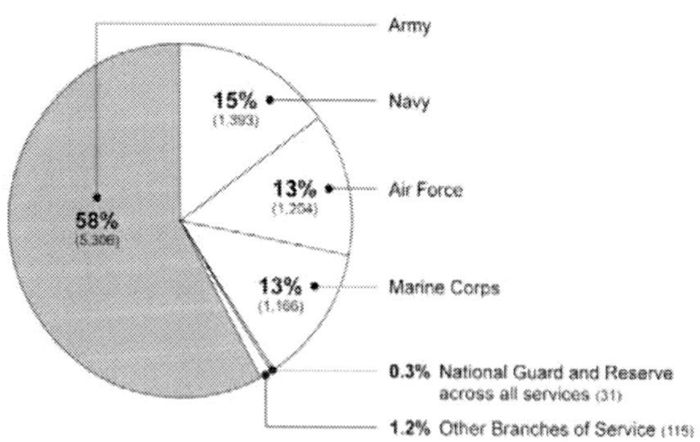

Source: GAO analysis of VA data.

Note: "Other" branches of service include the U.S. Coast Guard and Merchant Marines.

Figure 6. Independent Living Track Veterans during FY 2008-2011, by Branch of Service.

With regard to severity of service-connected disabilities, more than three-quarters of IL track veterans had a combined service-connected rating of at least 60 percent. Thirty-four percent of IL track veterans had a combined service-connected disability rating of 100 percent.[21] Many IL track veterans may have also been eligible for the VA Disability Compensation program's Individual Unemployability cash benefit.[22] Indeed, 38 percent of IL track veterans were eligible for this supplement to their disability compensation payments. Moreover, of those IL track veterans who were at least 60 years old, 85 percent had combined service-connected disability ratings of at least 60 percent and more than a third had combined ratings of 100 percent.

IL track veterans had a wide variety of service-connected disabilities, and most had more than one. Regardless of disability rating level, the most prevalent disabilities among this group were Post-traumatic Stress Disorder (PTSD), tinnitus ("ringing in the ears"), and hearing loss. As shown in figure 7, many of these disabilities—7 of the top 10 we identified in these cases—are similar to the most prevalent conditions among veterans rated by VA's Disability Compensation program in fiscal year 2011.

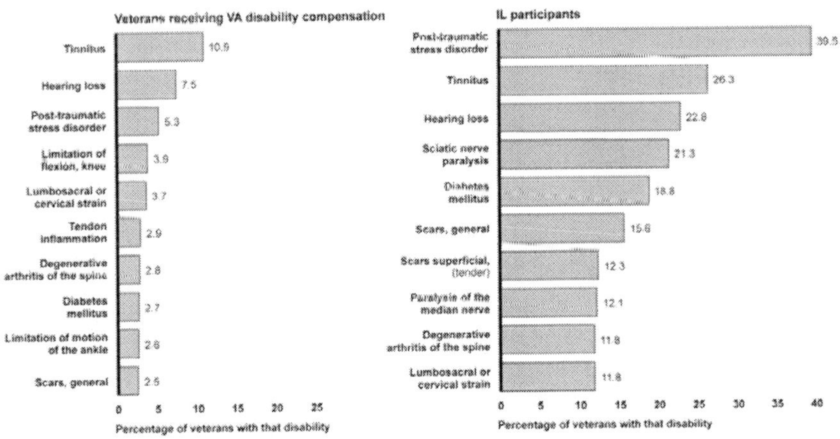

Source: GAO analysis of VA data.

Figure 7. Comparison of the 10 Most Prevalent Disabilities among Independent Living Track Veterans from FY 2008-2011 and Veterans Receiving Disability Compensation for FY 2011.

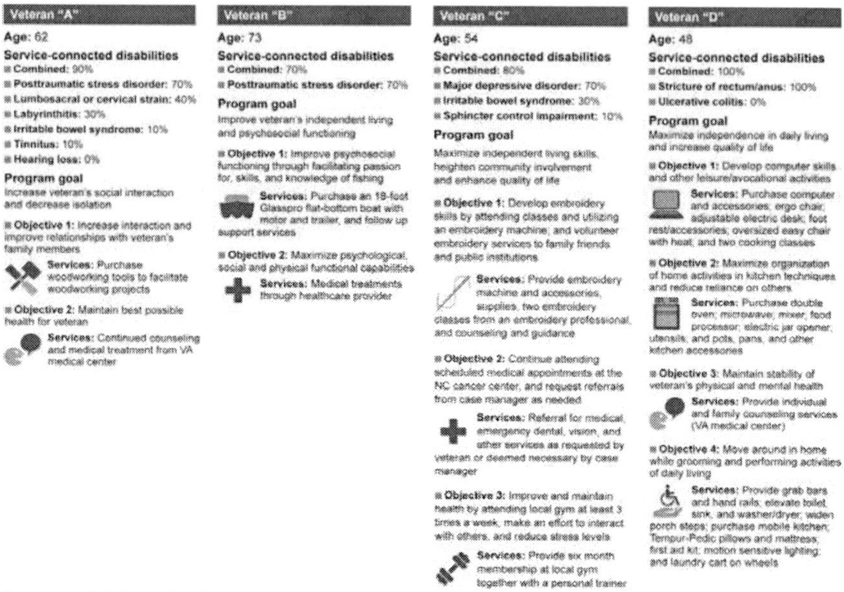

Source: GAO analysis of IL track veterans' case files from fiscal year 2008.

Figure 8. Examples of the Types of Goods and Services Provided in Four of the Independent Living Track Cases GAO Reviewed.

The IL Track Has Provided a Wide Range of Benefits

Our review of the case files of 182 randomly selected IL track veterans in fiscal year 2008 shows that they were provided a wide range of goods and services to help them live independently. Goods and services ranged from individual counseling and the installation of ramps to improve accessibility of veterans' homes, to a boat, camping gear, and computers intended by VA to help decrease veterans' social isolation. Figure 8 provides examples of the types of benefits provided in four IL track cases we reviewed. (See appendix III for a complete list of goods and services we identified in 182 IL track cases.) While VR&E can provide a wide range of benefits to IL track veterans, VR&E's policy as of November 2012 prohibits providing courses of study and training to veterans that would lead to academic degrees, and purchasing certain types of equipment, such as lawn tractors.[23] Our review of fiscal year 2008 IL cases shows instances where VR&E purchased lawn tractors and a riding mower. However, VR&E officials told us that there was no specific guidance prohibiting provision of such equipment in that year.

Table 1. Categories of Goods and Services Provided to Independent Living Track Veterans

Category	Category Definition	Examples
Adaptive equipment	Non-electronic goods that aid in independent living.	• Mattresses • Elastic shoelaces • Grab bars • Medication dispensers
Assistive devices and technology	Electronic goods used to improve veterans' functional capabilities.	• Lift chairs • Adjustable beds • Hydraulic patient lifter • Electric jar opener
Avocational/leisure equipment	Goods used for hobbies or recreational activities.	• Miter saw • Camping equipment • Boat • Silversmithing and engraving tools
Computer and camera equipment	Goods related to the purchase of a computer or camera.	• Laptops • Printers • Memory cards • Video camcorder
Counseling services	Social, vocational or psychotherapeutic services.	• Rehabilitation services • IL training • Adjustment counseling • Psychotherapy
Education and training	Education and training for "non-academic" purposes.	• Non-college egrees • Computer training • Apprenticeships • Driving lessons
Medical care and health-related services	Services to improve veterans' health.	• Dental care • Vision care • Gym memberships • Personal training
Residential adaptation and repair	Goods and services related to home remodeling, construction or repairs to enable veterans to access their homes more easily.	• Home construction • Ramp construction • Bath safety installations • Smoke detector
Other goods and services	Goods and services that we were unable to classify in one of the other categories listed.	• IL equipment • Boat shipping service • Warranties for goods and services purchased • Riding lawn mower/ tractors • Snow blowers

Source: GAO analysis of 182 case files of IL track veterans from fiscal year 2008.

As shown in table 1, we classified the wide range of goods and services we found in the 182 IL track case files we reviewed into nine general categories:

Although we were unable to estimate the number of times certain goods and services were provided in the 182 IL track cases we reviewed,[24] we generally found that the most common type of goods or services provided in the cases we reviewed were in three categories: 1) counseling, 2) education and training, and 3) computer and camera equipment.

We were, however, able to estimate the costs of the goods and services purchased for IL track cases. For all veterans who entered the IL track in fiscal year 2008, we estimate that VR&E purchased a total of almost $14 million in goods and services.[25] The average spent on purchases of goods and services per IL track case that year was nearly $6,000.[26] In the 182 IL track cases we reviewed, the total amount VR&E spent on purchases of goods and services per veteran varied from $20 to over $33,000. Nearly 40 percent of the 182 veterans received $4,000 or more on purchases of goods and services (see figure 9).

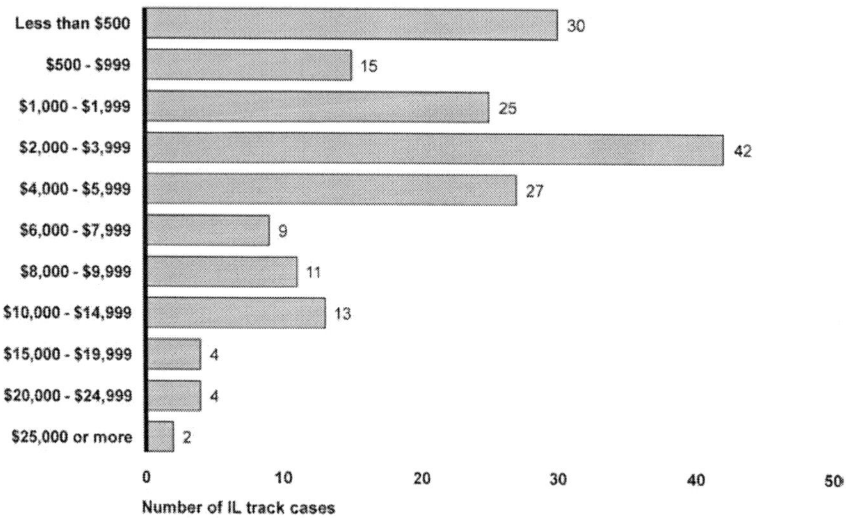

Source: GAO analysis of 182 case files of IL track veterans from fiscal year 2008.

Figure 9. Distribution of Independent Living Track Cases Reviewed by Costs of Goods and Services Purchased for Veterans.

MOST VETERANS COMPLETED "REHABILITATION" BUT WITH VARYING TIME FRAMES

Most Veterans in the IL Track are Ultimately Classified by VR&E as "Rehabilitated"

Based on our analysis of IL track veterans who began only one plan during fiscal year 2008, we found that most of these veterans were classified by VR&E as "rehabilitated"—successfully reaching and maintaining the goals identified in their IL plan.[27] By the end of fiscal year 2011, as shown in figure 10, about 89 percent of veterans who began an IL plan in fiscal year 2008 had been classified by VR&E as "rehabilitated." About 5 percent of cases were "discontinued" or closed by VR&E because the rehabilitation goals in the veteran's IL plan were not completed. The remaining 6 percent of veterans' cases were still open at the end of fiscal year 2011.

Of the 122 IL cases from fiscal year 2008 that had been discontinued, we found that about half were discontinued because the veteran declined benefits or did not respond when VA attempted to contact them. Another 29 percent were discontinued because the veteran died. Also, some VR&E officials and staff we spoke with during our site visits told us that veterans may drop out of the IL track for other reasons, such as their condition worsens or they experience family problems.

Furthermore, while most veterans were classified by VR&E as "rehabilitated," we found that the nature and complexity of IL plans can vary based on veterans' individual disabilities and needs. As such, some plans are easier for VR&E to close as rehabilitated than others. For example, in one case we reviewed, the IL plan for a veteran with rheumatoid arthritis only called for the purchase and installation of eight door levers and a grab rail for the bathtub, so that the veteran could enter the rooms of his home without pain or assistance, and be able to safely enter and exit the bathtub without fear of falling. Other cases were more complex to close as rehabilitated because of the nature of services being provided to the veteran. For instance, another case we reviewed called for providing a veteran who used a wheel-chair with medical, dental, and vision care as needed and about $24,000 in modifications to the veteran's home, including modifying the veteran's bathroom, widening doors and modifying thresholds, and installing an emergency exit ramp in a bedroom.

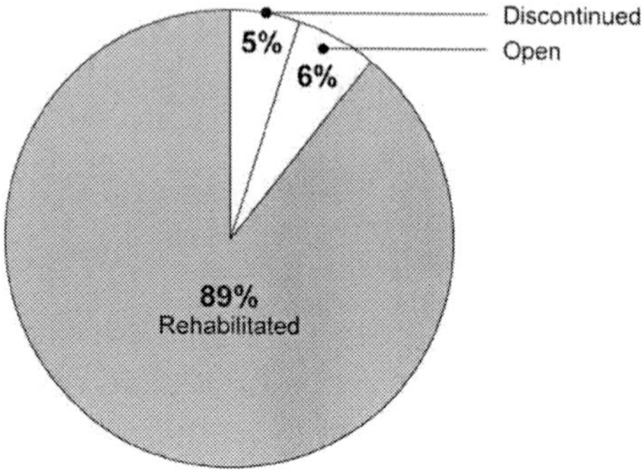

Source: GAO analysis of VA data.

Figure 10. Status at the End of FY 2011 of Independent Living Track Cases That Began in FY 2008.

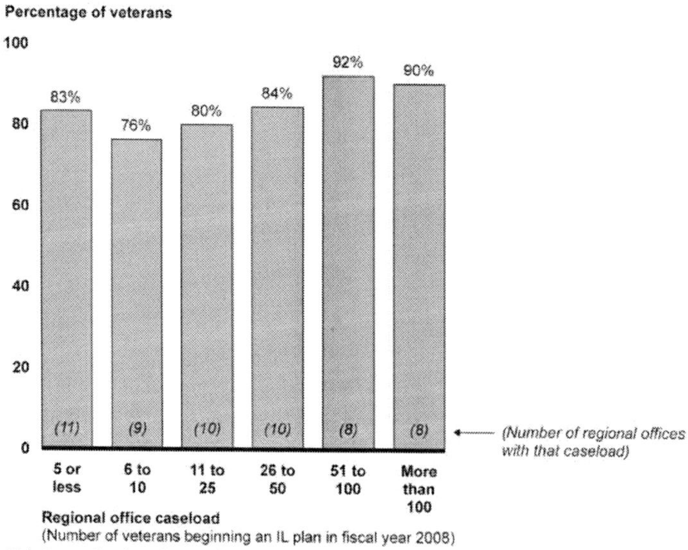

Source: GAO analysis of VA data.

Note: This table represents those veterans with only one IL plan who entered the IL track in fiscal year 2008 and who were rehabilitated by the end of fiscal year 2011.

Figure 11. Percentage of FY 2008 Independent Living Track Veterans Rehabilitated, by Regional Office Based on Caseload.

While the overall IL rehabilitation rate nationwide of 89 percent is fairly high, we found that the percentage of veterans who began an IL plan in fiscal year 2008 and were rehabilitated by the end of fiscal year 2011 varied by regional office.[28] IL rehabilitation rates in these cases ranged from 0[29] to 100 percent across regional offices, although about two-thirds of regional offices had rehabilitated 80 percent or more of 2008 IL track veterans by the end of fiscal year 2011. (See appendix IV for a complete list of rehabilitation rates for all regional offices.) In addition, VR&E's IL rehabilitation rate was higher in regional offices with larger IL caseloads. Among veterans who entered the IL track in fiscal year 2008, an average of 90 percent were rehabilitated at offices with more than 25 IL entrants, compared to an average of 79 percent at offices with 25 or fewer IL entrants (see figure 11).[30]

The Time to Rehabilitate IL Track Veterans Varied by Regional Office and Veteran Age

Furthermore, we found that fiscal year 2008 IL track veterans nationwide completed their IL plans, i.e., were classified rehabilitated, in an average of 384 days (about 13 months).[31] About 50 percent of these veterans completed their IL plans within 1 year, 79 percent within 2 years, and 88 percent within 3 years. Average days for these IL track veterans to complete their plans varied by regional office from a low of 150 days at the St. Paul Regional Office to a high of 895 days at the Roanoke Regional Office.[32] However, at most regional offices (49 of 53)[33] the average time to complete IL plans ranged from 226 to 621 days (8 to 21 months). (See appendix V for a complete list of rehabilitation times for all regional offices.) Also, as shown in figure 12, IL track veterans generally completed their plans in less time at regional offices with larger IL caseloads than at offices with smaller caseloads.

The average time for veterans to complete their IL plans also varied by veteran age. The oldest veterans completed their plans slightly more quickly than the youngest. More specifically, veterans who were 70 to 79 completed their plans in an average of 369 days, while those who were 20 to 29 completed them in an average of 413 days (see figure 13).[34]

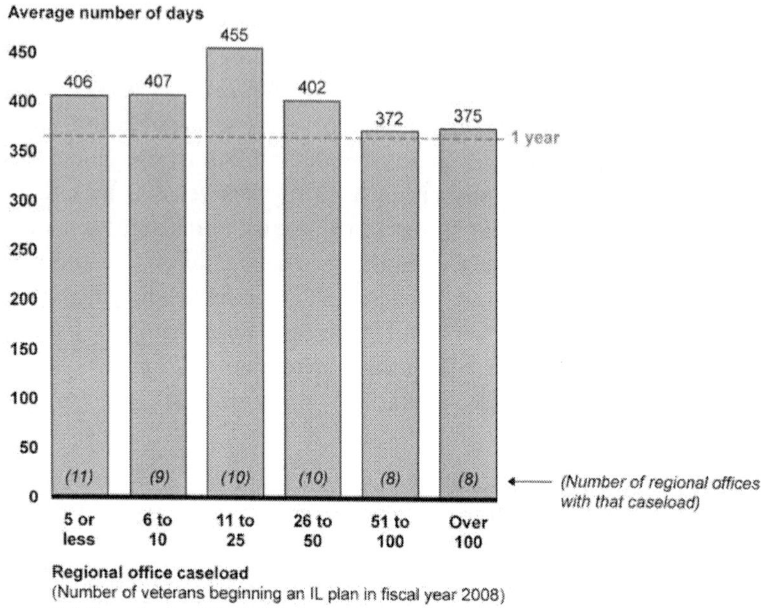

Source: GAO analysis of VA data.

Note: This table represents those veterans who began one IL plan in fiscal year 2008 and were rehabilitated by the end of fiscal year 2011.

Figure 12. Average Length of Time to Complete an Independent Living Plan, by Regional Office Based on Caseload.

GAO Analysis of Likelihood of Veterans Completing Their IL Plans

Because differences in the length of time to complete IL plans could have occurred by chance or be explained by many factors—including the type and severity of disability or veteran age—we used a statistical model to estimate the amount of time it would take certain groups of IL track veterans to complete their IL plans while controlling for type and severity of disability and other demographic characteristics.[35] (See appendix II for more detailed information on our model and analysis.) The results of our model showed that the chance of rehabilitation within 2 years varied by regional office. At four regional offices the chance of being rehabilitated within 2 years was less than 50 percent. At 18 offices the chance was between 50 and less than 90 percent. At 16 offices the chance was 90 percent or greater.

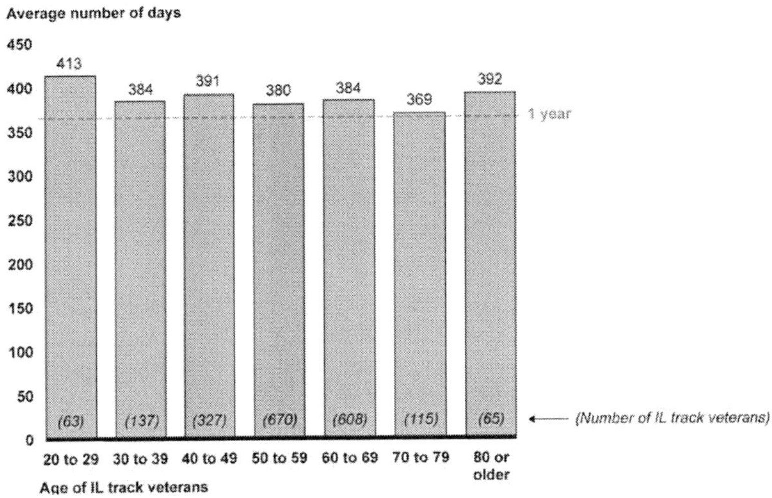

Source: GAO analysis of VA data.

Note: This table represents those veterans who began one IL plan in fiscal year 2008 and were rehabilitated by the end of fiscal year 2011.

Figure 13. Average Time to Complete Independent Living Plans, by Veteran Age Groups.

Our model also estimated that a veteran served by a regional office with a large IL caseload had a higher probability of completing an IL plan more quickly than a veteran served by an office with a small IL caseload. More specifically, we determined that a typical IL track veteran at an office with a total of 75 IL cases entering the IL track during fiscal years 2008 through 2011 had a 48 percent chance of completing an IL plan within 1 year and a 92 percent chance of completing an IL plan within 3 years,[36] while a veteran at a regional office with 700 IL cases had a 57 percent chance of completing an IL plan within 1 year and a 96 percent chance of completing their plan within 3 years (see figure 14).[37] Finally, based on our model we estimated that older veterans had a higher probability of completing an IL plan more quickly than younger veterans. For example, a 75 year old veteran had a 41 percent chance of completing an IL plan within one year, while a 30 year old veteran had a 33 percent chance. We found no meaningful differences in the time it takes to complete an IL plan as "rehabilitated" according to veteran gender and most disability types. However, we found small differences according to length of military service, education, and combined service-connected disability rating (see appendix II).

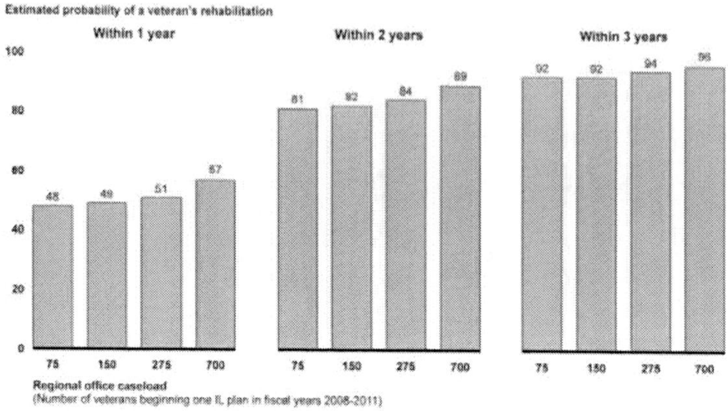

Source: GAO statistical analysis of VA data.

Note: Estimates were calculated from a statistical model. See appendix I and II for more information.

Figure 14. Estimated Probability of a Veteran Completing an Independent Living Plan within Certain Time Periods, by Regional Office Based on Caseload.

VR&E Exercises Limited Oversight of the IL Track

National oversight of VR&E's IL track is limited in four key areas: (1) ensuring compliance with case management requirements; (2) monitoring regional variation in IL track caseload and benefits provided; (3) adequacy of policies and procedures for approving expenditures on goods and services for IL track veterans; and (4) availability of critical program management information.

Regional Offices May Not Be Complying with VR&E Case Management Requirements

Based on VR&E's compliance reports from two of the regional offices we visited and interviews with staff in these offices, we found that some offices may not be complying with certain VR&E case management requirements governing the IL track. Specifically, some Vocational Rehabilitation Counselors (VRC) are not fulfilling VR&E's requirement to meet in-person each month with IL track veterans to monitor progress in completing their IL plans.[38] Site visit monitoring reports[39] from two regional offices we visited indicated that these offices faced difficulties complying with this requirement. According to these reports, some VRCs were not able to schedule monthly in-person meetings with IL track veterans to check their progress in completing their IL plans. In addition, VRCs we spoke with during our site visits said that compliance with this requirement continues to be a challenge due to the size of their caseloads and the distances that they have to travel to meet with veterans. While VR&E's Central Office acknowledges that it can be challenging for some offices to comply with this requirement, officials stated that face-to-face contact with IL track veterans is extremely important due to the nature of their disabilities and the need for more intensive rehabilitation services.[40]

Furthermore, while VR&E and VHA both have policies that require them to coordinate on the provision of goods and services for IL track veterans, we found that some VRCs experience challenges in doing so.[41] Specifically, VA regulations governing VR&E's IL track require that if a veteran needs special equipment and is eligible for such equipment under another VA program, the items will be provided under that program.[42] Therefore, prior to VR&E purchasing services for veterans, officials told us that VRCs are required to refer cases to other VA providers, such as VHA's Home Improvements and Structural Alterations (HISA) program and VA medical centers, to determine whether veterans are eligible to receive the goods and services identified in their plan from these providers. In addition, VHA 's policy directive for coordinating with VR&E is intended to ensure that all VR&E participants, including those in the IL track, receive timely access to VHA health care services. The directive requires medical center directors to (1) provide clinically appropriate care to VR&E participants, (2) establish procedures to manage these participants' timely access to care, and (3) ensure that clinical staff are trained in these procedures, including how to alert appropriate VBA officials when timeliness of care could be an issue, among other requirements.[43]

Despite these VR&E and VHA policies, our review of 182 IL track records found some instances where VR&E purchased goods and services that appear to be medically related, such as ramps and grab bars, and could have been provided by VHA. There may have been little coordination on IL track cases because, as VR&E officials and staff at the five VA regional offices we visited told us, coordinating with VHA medical center staff can be challenging. Several VRCs indicated that when they refer IL track cases to VHA physicians to determine whether any of the medical-related benefits identified in the IL plans—such as grab bars, wheelchairs, and safety rails—

had been or could be provided by VHA, in many instances, VHA physicians do not respond or respond too late. As a result, services for IL track veterans were either delayed or purchased by VR&E instead of VHA. According to some VHA staff, lack of or delays in coordination are sometimes due to differences in VR&E rehabilitation goals and VHA long-term medical goals for veterans. For example, VHA staff members mentioned they would not approve VRCs' requests for lift chairs unless veterans absolutely needed them because VHA staff members said their medical goal is to promote continued mobility.

VR&E Does Not Systematically Monitor Variation in IL Track Caseload Size and Benefits Provided

While IL track caseload size and benefits vary across regions, VR&E does not systematically monitor these variations. We found regional differences in the size of IL caseloads, the range of needs covered in a veteran's IL plan, and the types of goods and services provided. As shown in figure 15, the total IL track caseload during fiscal years 2008 through 2011 ranged from over 900 cases in the Montgomery Regional Office in Alabama to 4 cases in the Wilmington Regional Office in Delaware. (See appendix VI for annual IL caseload data.) While one would expect differences in caseload size based on the number of veterans in an office's service area, some differences in IL caseload could not be explained by the size of the veteran population in an office's service area. For example, while the estimated size of the veteran populations in Alabama and Massachusetts are similar, Montgomery's IL caseload of over 900 veterans was more than 100 times as large as Boston's IL caseload of 8 veterans. VR&E officials told us they are aware that some offices have low IL participation levels, and attributed some of the difference to factors, such as the presence of specialized treatment centers in certain areas of the county that can increase caseload numbers in those regions. However, evidence from our site visits suggests that there may be other factors that drive the number of veterans entering a region's IL track. For example, officials from the Detroit Regional Office—which had the second highest total IL caseload across fiscal years 2008 through 2011—attributed the size of their caseload to their office's focus on IL cases and community outreach efforts, including the involvement of veteran service organizations. The Atlanta Regional Office also mentioned that in addition to the size of the veteran population in Georgia and the presence of army bases, the size of their IL caseload is influenced by increased community interest in the IL track in recent years, and the informal efforts of past IL participants to provide information about the IL track to other veterans.

Based on discussions with regional personnel and our review of the results of past studies, IL plans and the goods and services provided can also vary by region. According to VR&E officials, the law gives VA broad discretion in defining the range of needs covered in an IL track plan, as well as in choosing the types of goods and services required to achieve the plan's goals. VR&E's policy does, however, prohibit the agency from providing courses of study and training leading to academic degrees, and purchasing certain types of equipment, such as lawn tractors. As a result, some regions appear to develop IL plans that address a broader range of needs while others elect to develop more focused plans. Officials we spoke with during our site visits also confirmed that regions differ in their approach to developing IL plans, and in one region, officials commented that some regions may develop simpler plans with fewer benefits to achieve VR&E's rehabilitation goal. Moreover, VR&E's 2008 study of the IL track reported that some regions relied repeatedly on the same types of benefits to meet veterans' IL needs.[44] For example, in the New York and Hartford regional offices, nearly 90 percent of IL participants were provided computer training. This was almost twice the rate of Detroit—the office with the next highest rate of providing veterans with computer training—in 44 percent of its IL cases. Other offices focused more heavily on providing goods or services to support veterans' avocational interests or on finding veterans volunteer opportunities, while some consistently focused on providing veterans with health club memberships. For example, the St. Petersburg Regional Office accounted for 33 percent of veterans receiving volunteer opportunities. In addition, the 2004 VR&E Task Force report noted significant differences in field office philosophy regarding the scope and administration of the IL track, and also recommended providing VR&E Central Office greater "line-of-site authority" over VR&E field operations.[45] As noted earlier, VBA's Office of Field Operations rather than VR&E's Central Office has direct line of authority over regional VR&E staff and operations.

While VA officials acknowledged the existence of regional variation in these areas, VR&E's current oversight approach may not be adequate to ensure consistent administration of the IL track across regions. The standards for internal control in the federal government emphasize the need for federal agencies to have timely information to effectively monitor and mitigate program risks.[46] To oversee administration of the IL track, VR&E has relied on the information provided through its general quality assurance (QA) activities and a series of periodic ad hoc studies. The QA activities are conducted by each region as well as VR&E's QA staff located in Nashville, Tennessee. However, these activities are limited in scope, frequency, and how the information is used. At the national level, a team of VR&E QA staff are required to perform periodic site visits to each VA regional office at least every 3 years, although officials told us they have not been able to meet this goal in recent years because of budgetary constraints. This team also periodically reviews a sample of veterans' records from VR&E's IL and employment tracks in selected regions. After each site visit and case review, the QA team produces a report for the particular region under review. While VR&E officials told us that QA results are "analyzed to determine trends," it is unclear how VR&E uses these results to ensure that consistent procedures are used by regional offices nationwide.

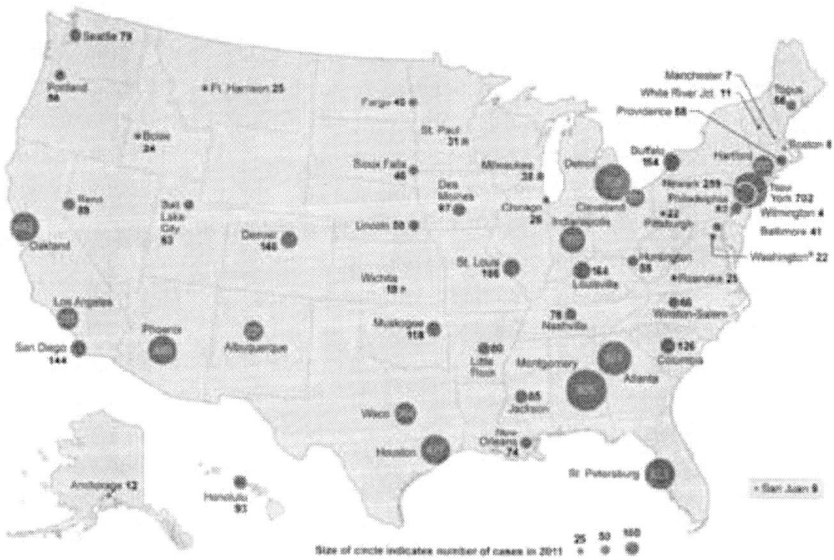

Source: GAO analysis of VA data.

[a] The Washington Regional Office, located in the District of Columbia, was recently designated the National Capital Region Benefits Office in November 2012.

Figure 15. The Vocational Rehabilitation and Employment Program's Overall Independent Living Caseload from FY 2008-2011, by Regional Office.

In addition to these QA activities, VA has funded two studies over the past several years on the VR&E program, including implementation of the IL track, and a third is under way.[47] In 2003, VA appointed a task force to evaluate the overall VR&E program and recommend ways service delivery could be improved. In 2008, as mentioned, a study was issued by VR&E on the types of services received by IL track participants and the impact those services had on veterans.[48] This study found, among other things, that IL participants received a broad range of services, and that some regional offices favored providing certain types of services to IL track veterans. Finally, in October 2012, VR&E awarded a contract for about $890,312 to study the IL track service delivery process, barriers and incentives for field staff when considering the provision of services, current and future training strategies, and other areas. VR&E officials anticipate receiving the final results from this study in July 2013.

VR&E Policy for Approving IL Track Expenditures Might Not Be Adequate

Considering the broad discretion VR&E provides to regions in determining the range of needs covered in IL track plans and the types of goods and services selected to meet these needs, VR&E's current policy for approving IL track expenditures may not be adequate. To guard against fraud, waste, abuse, and mismanagement, the standards for internal control emphasize the need for agencies to have appropriate levels of supervision and controls in place to prevent one individual from having responsibility for all key aspects of a transaction or event.[49] VR&E Central Office is responsible for managing the program's national budget. While officials told us that VRCs are required to include all cost estimates when they submit veterans' IL plans to be reviewed and approved by the region's VR&E Officer, VR&E was unable to provide any written policy or guidance that explicitly states this requirement for all IL expenditures.[50] VR&E's current written policies allow each region to unilaterally approve construction-related expenditures up to $25,000 per case and non-construction expenditures up to $100,000 per case without approval from VR&E Central Office. In addition, VRCs can spend up to $2,000 on construction-related expenditures and up to $25,000 on non-construction expenditures without supervisory review of any kind (see table 2). Under this policy, regional offices are permitted to purchase a broad range of items without any Central Office approval, resulting in some offices purchasing goods and services that may be questionable or that are costly. For example, in one of the 182 IL cases we reviewed, VR&E Central Office would not have been required to approve total expenditures of $18,829 for a riding lawn mower—which VR&E policy prohibits[51]—and other IL goods and services including a bed, bed frame, desktop computer, and woodworking equipment. In another case, VR&E Central Office approval would not have been required for the purchase of a boat, motor, trailer, and the boat's shipping cost to Molokai, Hawaii, among other items, totaling about $17,500.[52] Without appropriate approval levels, VR&E's IL track may be vulnerable to potential fraud, waste, and abuse.

VR&E Lacks Critical Information Needed for Oversight

VR&E does not collect or report critical program management information—such as the costs of goods and service purchased, the types of benefits provided, and the number of IL veterans served—that would help the agency in its oversight responsibilities. Specifically, VR&E's Corporate WINRS case management system—commonly referred to as "CWINRS"—lacks information on the total amount of funds VR&E expends on IL benefits because the agency does not maintain specific cost information on each of its five tracks or the key program areas these tracks represent, which are employment services and independent living. VR&E aggregates costs across all its tracks, despite VA's managerial cost accounting policies that require the costs of products and services to be captured for management purposes.[53] Federal financial accounting standards also recommend that costs of programs be measured and reported.[54] According to officials, they do not collect cost information on the IL track alone because they view the five tracks as a single program with the same overarching goal—to help veterans achieve their employment goals. However, in our 2009 report on the VR&E program,[55] we reported that VR&E serves veterans with fundamentally different program goals and outcomes—those seeking to obtain employment and those seeking to live independently.[56] As a result, we recommended that VR&E separately track its IL rehabilitation rate.

In addition, the CWINRS system does not collect information on the types of IL benefits provided to veterans in a standardized manner that can be easily aggregated and analyzed for oversight purposes. Currently, VRCs are required to write in a description of the benefits they purchased for IL track veterans in CWINRS. We found, however, that the recorded descriptions lack consistency and vary in their level of detail. In several of the IL track cases we reviewed, the goods and services purchased were grouped together under a general description, such as "IL equipment" or "IL supplies," without any further details. In other cases, VRCs recorded each purchase separately. For instance, in one case, the VRC created separate entries for each item purchased, for example, "desktop computer," "computer desk," "Queen Mattress," "all in one printer," "USB cable and ink," "threshold ramp," and "washer." In addition, we found that controls for data entry are not adequate to ensure that all important data is recorded.[57] For example, we estimated that the service provider field was either missing or unclear for one or more services in about 15 percent of all IL cases that began in fiscal year 2008. Moreover, in another 7 percent of IL cases that began during fiscal year 2008, we found that service provider data was unavailable because CWINRS had overwritten veterans' 2008 IL plans with subsequent plans. CWINRS only retains veterans' current IL plan.[58]

Furthermore, CWINRS does not provide VR&E with the information it needs to account for the actual number of IL track veterans it serves to monitor its statutory entrant cap and program operations. The law allows VR&E to initiate "programs" of independent living services and assistance for no more than a specified number of veterans each year, which is currently set at 2,700.[59] A VR&E policy letter to VA regional offices, dated December 14, 2010, states that "VR&E Service will monitor new IL programs by tracking the number of veterans entering independent living case status in each fiscal year and notify the field of any necessary action if the 2,700 statutory limit is being approached."[60] However, in analyzing VR&E's administrative data, we found that VR&E counts the number of IL plans developed annually and not the number of individual veterans admitted to the track. VR&E officials told us that the law does not limit the number of IL plans that can be developed for a veteran in a single fiscal year.[61] Because multiple IL plans can be developed for an individual veteran during the same fiscal year, veterans with multiple plans are counted more than once towards the statutory cap by CWINRS. Based on data from CWINRS, 403 (4 percent) of the 9,215 veterans beginning an IL plan during fiscal years 2008 through 2011 had more than one plan during that time. About 22 percent of these veterans had more than one IL plan in the same fiscal year. From fiscal years 2008 through 2011, VR&E did not exceed the statutory cap (see figure 16).

Table 2. Level of Approval Required for Construction and Non-Construction-Related Expenditures in Independent Living Track Cases

Required level of approval	Construction-related expenditures	Non-construction related expenditures
No supervisory approval required[a]	Less than $2,000	Less than $25,000
Regional VR&E Officer		$25,000 to less than $75,000
Regional Office Director	$2,000 through $25,000	$75,000 through $100,000
VR&E Central Office	More than $25,000	More than $100,000

Source: GAO analysis of VA policies.

[a] VR&E officials told us that all IL plans require supervisory review. However, VR&E's written policies do not require IL expenditures to be reviewed and approved by the VR&E officer unless they meet certain cost-thresholds.

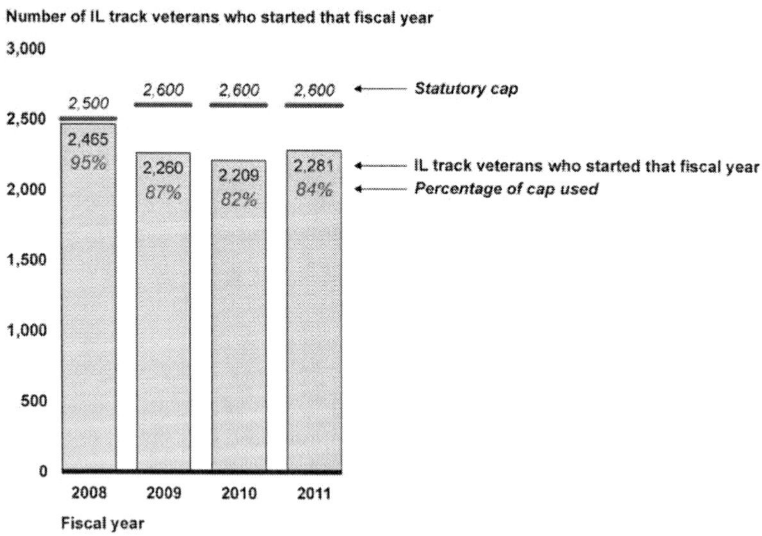

Source: GAO analysis of VA data.

Figure 16. Number of and Statutory Cap on Veterans Entering the Independent Living Track from FY 2008-2011.

Moreover, VR&E officials indicated that they were unaware that CWINRS was calculating the number of plans and not individual veterans. As a result, VR&E lacks complete information on the number of veterans it is serving through the IL track at any given time—information it could use to better manage staff, workloads, and program resources. According to the standards for internal control, it is important for program managers to have reliable and timely "operational" information to ensure agency goals are met, resources are used efficiently and effectively, and requirements under various laws and regulations are being complied with.[62]

Finally, recent evaluations of CWINRS have determined that the system does not meet VR&E's current needs and limits its oversight abilities because important data elements are not captured to support the agency's "evolving business needs."[63] According to a 2012 VR&E report, VR&E plans to improve CWINRS by (1) increasing data automation to reduce instances of human error, and (2) enhancing system controls to improve the accuracy and comprehensiveness of the data, among other improvements. However, it appears that the CWINRS redesign will not enable VR&E to obtain data on IL track expenditures from the system or to use the system to accurately and efficiently track the types of goods and services the IL track provides. While officials told us that they plan to modify the system to enable them to track individual veterans served through the IL track, they could provide no time frame for this project and noted that it could take up to 3 years to obtain funding for it.

CONCLUSION

VR&E's IL track can provide a wide range of benefits to help veterans with service-connected disabilities maximize their ability to live independently when the achievement of an employment goal is not currently feasible. Under the law, each VA region has broad discretion in determining the range and types of goods and services each IL track veteran should receive. Consequently, adequate oversight at the national level is extremely important in ensuring that IL track case management requirements are met, the track is administered consistently across regions, expenditures for goods and services are appropriate, and critical IL track information is collected and used.

In this context and absent better coordination with VHA, VR&E will continue to face challenges in ensuring goods and services for IL track veterans are provided by VHA, when appropriate, in a timely manner. With regard to VR&E's Central Office oversight, its current policy governing the review and approval of expenditures might not effectively mitigate the risk of fraud, waste, abuse, or mismanagement inherent in activities, such as the development and implementation of IL plans, where there are few limitations on the types and cost of goods and services that can be provided. Furthermore, without collecting information on cost and the types of benefits regional offices provide to IL track veterans, and maintaining an information system that ensures IL track data are recorded consistently and are accurate and complete, VR&E cannot effectively oversee the performance and activities of its IL track. Finally, as more servicemembers from the conflicts in Iraq and Afghanistan transition into civilian life and veterans' programs and as the overall veteran population ages, the demand for IL services will likely increase. VR&E must, therefore, be able to accurately count the number of individual IL track veterans served to ensure it can effectively manage its cap and assess program performance and resource needs.

Recommendations for Executive Action

The Secretary of Veterans Affairs should direct the Undersecretary for Benefits to take the following actions:

1. Work with the Undersecretary for Health to explore options on ways to enhance coordination to ensure IL track veterans' needs are met by VHA, when appropriate, in a timely manner. This could include improving staff education, response times to IL referrals, and the provision of medically related goods and services.
2. Implement an oversight approach that enables VR&E to better ensure consistent administration of the IL track across regions. In developing this approach, consider ensuring that VR&E's CWINRS system:
    - Tracks the total cost and types of benefits provided to each veteran in the IL track by regional office.
    - Accounts for the number of individual veterans served to ensure that the agency has the information it needs to adequately manage the IL track.
    - Contains stronger data entry controls to ensure that IL track information is recorded in a consistent manner and is accurate and complete.
3. Reassess and consider enhancing the agency's current policy concerning the required level of approval for IL track expenditures, given the broad discretion individual regional offices have in determining the types of goods and services IL track veterans receive.

Agency Comments and Our Evaluation

We provided a draft of this report to the Secretary of Veterans Affairs for review and comment. VA generally agreed with our conclusions, and concurred with our three recommendations. In addition, VA provided technical comments that we have incorporated in the report where appropriate. With regards to our recommendation that VA enhance coordination between VR&E and VHA on the provision of IL benefits to veterans, VA noted there are efforts underway that will permit VR&E counselors to make IL referrals to VHA providers through VHA's Compensation and Pension Record Interchange system, also referred to as CAPRI. In addition to these efforts, we encourage VR&E and VHA to continue to explore other options to enhance coordination, such as engaging in staff education and training efforts to improve the timely provision of IL benefits and prevent any duplication. Furthermore, with regards to our recommendation to improve IL track oversight, VA said that it will perform an assessment of its current IL track oversight procedures and consider including enhancements to CWINRS. Because having a sound information system plays such a critical role in helping program managers monitor agency performance and operations, we urge VA to take steps to prioritize enhancements to CWINRS. Finally, VA noted that, in response to our recommendation that it reassess its current policy for approving IL track expenditures, it plans to make any needed improvements by March 2014. As part of its assessment process, we believe that VA should review its existing cost-thresholds for approving all IL expenditures, including non-construction related expenditures, to ensure adequate oversight of goods and services purchased for veterans.

Daniel Bertoni
Director, Education, Workforce,
and Income Security Issues

Appendix I: Objectives, Scope, and Methodology

The objectives of this report were to examine (1) the characteristics of veterans who have participated in the IL track, as well as the types and costs of benefits they were provided; (2) the extent to which their independent living plans were completed, and the time it took; and (3) the extent to which the IL track has been administered appropriately and consistently.

To answer these objectives, we used a variety of methodologies, which are described in greater detail below. Specifically, we analyzed VA administrative data from fiscal years 2008 through 2011 to provide information on the characteristics and outcomes of veterans who participate in the IL track, and how long it takes to achieve these outcomes. We also used statistical models to determine any differences in rehabilitation times. In addition, to determine the types of benefits provided and their costs, we conducted a case file review of a random, generalizable sample of 182 veterans who started in the IL track during fiscal year 2008. Lastly, to examine the administration of the IL track, we visited five VA regional offices and interviewed officials and staff from VR&E, Specially Adapted Housing (SAH), Prosthetics and Sensory Aid Service (PSAS) under the Veterans Health Administration (VHA), and veteran service organizations. We also reviewed relevant federal laws and regulations, standards for internal controls and managerial cost accounting, as well as VR&E policies, procedures, and other relevant studies and documentation.

Analysis of VA Administrative Data

We analyzed VA administrative data in the Corporate WINRS system—commonly referred to as "CWINRS"—from fiscal years 2008 through 2011 to describe the characteristics and outcomes of veterans in the IL track, and how long it takes veterans to achieve these outcomes.[64]

We began our analysis in fiscal year 2008 because officials told us the data was not reliable in previous years and modifications were made to improve its reliability in fiscal year 2007. We assessed the reliability of the data by performing electronic testing, reviewing existing documentation, and interviewing knowledgeable agency officials. Based on these efforts, we found the data to be sufficiently reliable for our purpose, unless otherwise noted.

To identify our universe of 9,215 veterans who started in the IL track during fiscal years 2008 through 2011, we counted the number of individual veterans who had an "IL status" recorded in CWINRS during our time frame.[65] While veterans can enter into the IL track more than once in a given fiscal year, we counted a veteran only once if he or she had more than one IL status during these years. To determine the characteristics of the 9,215 veterans who began in the IL track during fiscal years 2008 through 2011, we examined several demographic variables in CWINRS, including veterans' age, gender, types of disabilities, and combined disability rating. Data on the war era in which veterans served was obtained from VA's Benefits Delivery Network.

To examine the outcomes of veterans in the IL track, we limited our analysis to veterans who began only one IL plan at some point during fiscal year 2008. This accounted for about 92 percent of the 2,465 veterans who began an IL plan during fiscal year 2008. The remaining 8 percent of veterans who had more than one plan were excluded from our analysis because of potential data reliability issues associated with how certain case actions were recorded. In our analysis of IL veteran rehabilitation rates, we excluded veterans whose cases were transferred to one of VR&E's employment tracks.

To estimate the difference in rehabilitation times across regional offices and groups of veterans with various characteristics, we used different statistical models. These "survival modeling" methods allowed us to appropriately estimate rehabilitation probabilities at various points in an IL plan, even when a significant proportion of the cases are discontinued or in progress. Our models used the same VA administrative data noted above for veterans in the IL track who began only one IL plan at some point during fiscal years 2008 through 2011. Consequently, our model results only apply to a subset of veterans, which make up about 95 percent of the veterans who began in the IL track during this time frame. For a detailed discussion of our statistical models, see appendix II.

Analysis of IL Veteran Cases

To obtain information on the types of benefits provided through the IL track, as well as the costs and coordination of these benefits, we conducted a case file review of a random, generalizable sample of 182 veterans whose cases started in the IL track at some point during fiscal year 2008. To track and manage IL cases, VR&E utilizes both paper records located at each regional office, and electronic case records in the CWINRS system. For the purpose of our file review, we used veterans' electronic records in CWINRS, and found the information in these records to be sufficient for our purpose.[66] We selected fiscal year 2008 because it allowed us to follow veterans' progress in the IL track beyond 24 months—the authorized benefit duration time frame unless a 6-month extension is approved.

We stratified our sample of 182 cases into three groups—those veterans' whose cases were (1) rehabilitated, (2) discontinued, or (3) still open.[67] We used this approach to obtain information on any differences in IL benefits and expenditures by veteran groups. We also elected to use a sample design that mixes the features of a proportional allocation and equal sample per stratum. Table 3 provides more detailed information on our sample stratification.

To produce population estimates from our sample of cases, information collected from each case reviewed was weighted in the analysis to account statistically for the total population of all IL track cases started in fiscal year 2008. Because our estimates for the entire population of IL track cases that started in fiscal year 2008 are based on a probability sample of these cases, they are subject to sampling error. To recognize the possibility that other samples drawn from this population might yield different results, we express our confidence in the precision of our sample's results as a 95 percent confidence interval. A 95 percent confidence interval is expected to include the actual value for the population in 95 out of 100 samples drawn from the population. With regard to expenditures in IL track cases, at the 95 percent confidence interval, the amount of total expenditures across all IL track cases that started in fiscal year 2008 falls between $11.3 million and $16.6 million; the actual amount expended, on average, in these cases falls between $4,835 and $7,104.

To conduct our case file review, we developed a web-based data collection instrument to record information from the electronic printouts VR&E provided us with of veterans' records. After these records were collected, GAO staff members entered the information into the electronic data collection instrument for each veteran case in our sample. Once the data was entered, a second GAO staff member reviewed each entry for clarity and accuracy. With regard to the types of benefits provided to IL track veterans, we cannot generalize the types of goods and services provided because we recorded in our data collection instrument information on only eight goods and services identified in each of the 182 IL case files we reviewed. However, we were able to generalize information we obtained on IL track service providers from the IL cases we reviewed because in less than 3 percent of these cases, there were at least eight service providers. Our estimate of the number of cases where service provider information was missing, unclear, or overwritten in CWINRS may be slightly understated. The 95 percent confidence interval for the 15 percent of cases where the service provider information was unclear or missing for one or more service ranged from 9 to 21 percent. The 95 percent confidence interval for the 7 percent of cases we reviewed where one or more service was overwritten in CWINRS ranged from 4 to 11 percent.

Table 3. Size of Sample of Independent Living Track Cases, by Strata and Proportion of Population

Sample strata	Number of Cases
Rehabilitated cases	88
Discontinued cases	47
Open cases	47
Total	**182**

Source: GAO analysis of VA data.

Regional Site Visits and Agency Interviews

To better understand the extent to which the IL track is being effectively administered, we visited five VA regional offices—San Diego, California; Atlanta, Georgia; Detroit, Michigan; Philadelphia, Pennsylvania; and the District of Columbia.[68] We selected these sites because they were geographically diverse, and have varying levels of IL track participation and success in achieving VR&E's IL rehabilitation goal. During each of our site visits, we interviewed VR&E Officers and vocational rehabilitation counselors (VRCs) using a standard set of questions to identify how IL cases were managed and any factors that may have affected the administration of the IL track. In particular, during our Detroit and Atlanta site visits, we interviewed VRCs who specialized in working on IL cases. Moreover, we obtained the perspectives of veteran service organizations that work with IL track veterans at two regional offices we visited—Detroit and Atlanta. Furthermore, we interviewed SAH and PSAS officials at the national level and relied on our case file review to determine the extent to which the IL track cases were referred to VA and non-VA service providers. In addition, we interviewed SAH and PSAS staff during our site visits to determine the extent to which VR&E, SAH, and PSAS coordinate in the provision of goods and services to IL track veterans.

Appendix II: Statistical Analysis of Independent Living Plan Rehabilitation Times

We used statistical models to estimate the difference in rehabilitation times across regional offices and groups of veterans with various characteristics. These "survival modeling" methods can appropriately estimate rehabilitation probabilities at various points in an IL plan, even when a significant proportion of the cases are discontinued or in progress. In addition, survival methods allowed us to estimate the unique association between rehabilitation times and various other factors, described below. In this appendix, we describe the data we used to fit the models and their structure, assumptions, and estimates.

We estimated our models using VA administrative data on veterans who began exactly one IL plan from fiscal years 2008 through 2011. Due to the data reliability issues described in appendix I, our analysis excluded veterans who began multiple IL plans during this period. Consequently, our results only apply to this subset of 8,737 veterans, who made up 94.8 percent of the original population.

[69] We measured the length of time each veteran spent in his or her IL plan as the duration between the start of the plan and one of three later times: entering rehabilitation status, discontinuing the plan, or being in progress on September 30, 2011, the end of our observation period. We modeled rehabilitation as the outcome of interest, treating discontinued or in progress plans as having rehabilitation times that were censored. Among the veterans starting IL plans from fiscal years 2008 through 2011, 3.2 percent discontinued their IL plans prior to rehabilitation, and 35.9 percent had plans that were in progress on September 30, 2011. These data imply that 91.7 percent of the censored observations were in-progress cases, which suggests that most of the censoring is likely to be uninformative. We found no large differences in the probability of dropping out of an IL plan across the covariates we included in our models.

Model Structure and Assumptions

We fit the data to several types of Cox proportional hazards models. The primary model took the following form:

$$\lambda_{ij}(\mathrm{t}) = \lambda_{0j}(\mathrm{t}) \exp(x_{ij}\beta)$$

$\lambda_{ij}(\mathrm{t})$ denotes the hazard rate of rehabilitation at time t after veteran i enters an IL plan, and $\lambda_{0j}(\mathrm{t})$ denotes the baseline hazard rate for the reference veteran with covariates equal to zero, served by one of j = 1, 2, … ,36 regional offices. We combined a number of offices that served less than 50 veterans into a residual group, in order to ensure sufficient sample within each office. The sample sizes within offices ranged from 58 to 908. x_{ij} is a vector of the following covariates: age, length of military service, and indicators for sex, branch of service, era of service, education, year the IL plan began, partial vs. full disability,[70] and disability type.[71] We coded the covariates such that the baseline reference veteran was substantively meaningful—a male Army veteran with a high school education, who served in the Vietnam era, entered an IL plan in fiscal year 2008, was processed by the Detroit Regional Office, and had a full musculoskeletal disability—either by setting values of categorical variables to the appropriate levels or by centering continuous variables at their means. All categorical variables included levels for missing data.

In this application, the proportional hazard structure of the model implies that the instantaneous rate of rehabilitation at any time during an IL plan, or the hazard, varies across values of the covariates by a constant amount over time. For example, the model assumes that rehabilitation rates vary by the same amounts among veterans with different types of disabilities after 12 months, 18 months, or any other point in an IL plan. In our initial exploratory data analysis, Kaplan-Meier estimates of the hazard and survival functions suggested that the hazard was not proportional across regional offices. Using an unstratified version of the model above that included fixed effects for regional offices, we found that the Schoenfeld residuals for many offices were correlated with time at a sufficiently high level to reject the hypothesis that the hazard functions were proportional across the covariates ($p < .0001$).[72] These results are consistent with our interviews and document reviews suggesting that program administration varied across offices, which could produce variation in hazard functions. (The body of this report summarizes these administrative inconsistencies in more detail.) For these reasons, we stratified the baseline hazard function by regional office, and we used this version of the model to calculate hazard rate ratios and elasticities, along with their standard errors, in table 3. Under the stratified model, we failed to reject the proportional hazards assumption for $\alpha < .47$.

The estimated rehabilitation (failure) probabilities discussed in the body of this report came from a version of the model that did not stratify by office and, instead, assumed office fixed effects. This allowed us to calculate illustrative rehabilitation probabilities by various follow-up points and for specific covariate values, without having to produce 36 sets of estimates implied by separate hazard functions for each office. The differences in the estimated probabilities across covariate values should resemble estimates that we would have calculated from the stratified model, because estimates of β and their variances were similar in both versions. The hazard rate ratios and elasticities in table 3 are consistent with our estimated rehabilitation probabilities in the body of the report. To calculate these probabilities, we fixed the value of each covariate at its sample mode or mean, depending on whether the variable was categorical or continuous. For this profile of covariate values, we calculated survival probabilities at various times using the estimated parameters of the unstratified model, and transformed them to failure probabilities by subtracting the survival estimates from 1.

Table 4. Estimates from Cox Hazard Model of Time Spent in Independent Living Plans, among Veterans Starting a Plan in FY 2008-2011

Variable	Hazard ratio	Standard error	Pr(Hazard ratio = 1)	95% Lower bound	95% Upper bound
Age (years)		0.0022	0.005	1.0019	1.0106
Length of service (years)		0.0026	0.012	1.0014	1.0117
Era of service					
Vietnam (Reference Group)					
Gulf War		0.0572	0.505	0.9312	1.1559
Global War on Terror		0.0735	0.174	0.9605	1.2495
Korea		0.0869	0.835	0.8611	1.2033
Peacetime		0.0453	0.499	0.8841	1.0618
World War II		0.0956	0.164	0.6876	1.0654
Education					
High school (Reference Group)					
Less than high school		0.0773	0.379	0.7897	1.0940
Some college		0.0339	0.507	0.9129	1.0461
College		0.0486	0.090	0.8232	1.0142
Graduate		0.1224	0.207	0.9280	1.4111
Missing data		0.0501	0.000	1.0790	1.2757
Sex					
Male (reference group)					
Female		0.0527	0.950	0.8985	1.1056
Missing data		0.1184	0.565	0.7238	1.1929
Branch of service					
Army (reference group)					
Air Force		0.0410	0.047	0.8377	0.9987
Coast Guard / other		0.1173	0.995	0.7953	1.2591
Marines		0.0463	0.425	0.9494	1.1311
Navy		0.0400	0.397	0.8902	1.0472
Year entered IL plan					
2008 (reference group)					

Variable		Standard error	Pr(Hazard ratio = 1)	95% Lower bound	95% Upper bound
2009		0.0312	0.001	0.8319	0.9543
2010		0.0306	0.000	0.7272	0.8473
2011		0.0485	0.000	0.6887	0.8793
Severity of disability					
Combined rating of 100 (reference group)					
Combined rating less than 100		0.0342	0.004	1.0299	1.1638
PT/missing data		0.0806	0.023	0.6515	0.9694
Type of disability					
Dental and oral		0.0999	0.665	0.8638	1.2578
conditions					
Gynecological conditions and Disorders of the breast		0.0883	0.580	0.7916	1.1397
Infectious diseases, immune Disorders and nutritional Deficiencies		0.0792	0.629	0.8177	1.1294
Muscle injuries		0.0666	0.755	0.8981	1.1598
Neurological conditions and Convulsive disorders		0.0375	0.540	0.9059	1.0531
Other sense organs		0.2290	0.606	0.5225	1.4602
The cardiovascular system		0.0343	0.069	0.8705	1.0053
The digestive system		0.0352	0.083	0.8702	1.0085
The ear		0.0334	0.742	0.9475	1.0786
The endocrine system		0.0447	0.017	1.0173	1.1926
The eye		0.0495	0.509	0.8745	1.0688
The genitourinary system		0.0362	0.294	0.8928	1.0349
The hemic and lymphatic systems		0.1385	0.261	0.9038	1.4518
The musculoskeletal system		0.0310	0.115	0.8909	1.0126
The respiratory system		0.0427	0.950	0.9171	1.0845
The skin		0.0314	0.612	0.9243	1.0474
VA regional office strata included					

Source: GAO statistical analysis of VA administrative data.

Note: N = 8,655, with 5,252 failures. Estimates of "hazard ratios" are exponentiated coefficients from a Cox hazard model, with reference groups as indicated. For the continuous covariates, age and length of service, the entries imply elasticities. For the disability type covariates, the entries represent the proportional change in the hazard of completing an IL plan for a veteran who has the listed disability, compared to a veteran who does not have the disability. (The disability types are not mutually exclusive and exhaustive groups, because veterans can have more than one type of disability.)

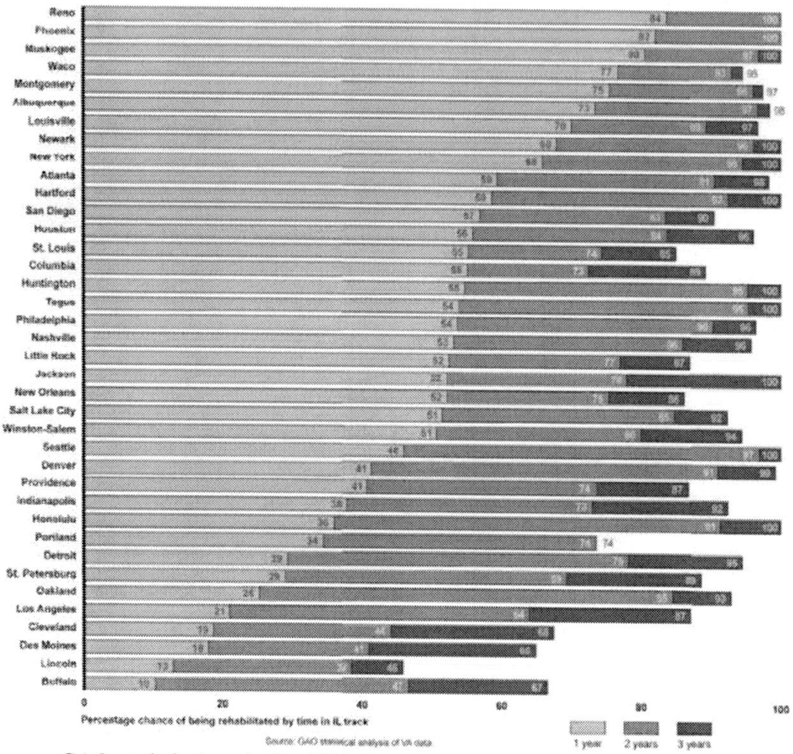

Source: GAO statistical analysis of VA data.

Note: We did not estimate the probability of a veteran being rehabilitated at regional offices where fewer than 50 veterans began IL plans during fiscal years 2008 through 2011.

Figure 17. Multivariate Failure Function Estimates from a Cox Hazard Model of Time Spent in Independent Living Plans, FY 2008-2011.

We estimated a final version of the model that used neither office strata nor fixed effects. This allowed us to estimate the association between office workload, measured by the total number of IL plans developed from fiscal year 2008 through 2011, and rehabilitation timeliness. Stratifying the model by office or estimating fixed effects would have absorbed the variation needed to estimate the coefficient on workload, as an office-level covariate.

Results

Table 3 provides estimates of β and hazard ratios derived from them, along with standard errors and p values for the hypothesis that each ratio equals 1. These estimates come from the stratified model above. Figure 17 presents the failure functions implied by the separate hazard functions the model assumes for each regional office. These results are generally consistent with those discussed in the body of this report, where we interpret the results in more detail.

APPENDIX III: LIST OF GOODS AND SERVICES PROVIDED TO SAMPLE OF INDEPENDENT LIVING TRACK VETERANS FROM OUR CASE FILE REVIEW

The table below lists the goods and services as they were recorded in the 182 cases we reviewed in the CWINRS system.

Goods and Services Provided	Frequency
Counseling Services	
"(1) Specialized Contractial Counseling Services 637"	5
"(1) Specialized Contractual Counseling"	1
"(1) Specialized Contractual Counseling Services 637, Vocational, Educational, Psychological or Personal adjustment counseling which I"	3
"(1) Specialized Independent Living Services 638"	1
"(1) Specialized Rehabilitation Service 631"	9
"(1) Specialized Rehabilitation Services"	6
"(1) Specialized Rehabilitation Services 631, Specialized services involving unique skills and techniques, such as learning di"	3
"(1) Specialized contractual counseling services 637; IILP Initial Assessment"	1
"(1)Special contractual Counseling"	1
"(316) Contract Counseling Assistance 451"	1
"(339) Special Services 532"	1
"(343) Rehab SErvices 556"	13
"(343) Rehab Services"	1
"(343) Rehab Services 556, All services not otherwise described to advance the objectives of the rehabilita"	9
"(343) Rehab Services 556; Connections Vocational Services; IILP Evals; All service not otherwise described to advance the objectives of the rehabilita"	2

(Continued)

Goods and Services Provided	Frequency
"(372) Independent Living Services 644, Provide Independent Living services (i.e. IL Evaluation, Occupational Therapy Ev"	1
"(372) Psychotherapy 667; provide psychotherapy and adjustment counseling"	4
"Adjustment Counseling 113"	1
"Rehab Services"	5
"Rehabilitation Counseling Services 158, Specialized counseling services as required to assist and support veteran in ful"	1
"SRS/IL Special Rehab Service/Independen Li"	29
"SRS/V Special Rehab Service/Vocaational; Center for Independent Living; IL Case Mgmt"	1
"SRS/V Special Rehab Service/Vocational"	31
"Special Rehab Service/Independent Living"	7
"Special Rehab. Srvs/Indepen. Living 24"	1
"Special Services."	1
"Special rehab service/Independent Living"	1
"Specialized Counseling Services 176"	1
Medical Care and Health Related Services	
"Cora Coleman Senior Center; 9 month swim membership"	1
"Dr. Sandoval; Eye exam"	1
"Exercise gym membership"	1
"Express Healthcare"	1
"Gym Membership-6 Months"	1
"Medical ID bracelet purchase and delivery"	1
"Medical care; SRS/M Special Rehab Services/Medical"	1
"Medical, Dental, Vision / Related Services 169, Comprehensive evaluation of medical, dental, or vision difficulties and provisio"	3
"Milwaukee VA Medical Center"	2
"Personal Trainig Session-Master Level"	1
"Personal Training - 24 Sessions"	1
"Providence; yoga membership fees -initial"	1
"Senior gym membership, and seniro swim membership"	1
"SRS/M Special Rehab Service/Medical"	40
"The Providence Institute; yoga class"	1
"VA MEDICAL CENTER -ANN ARBOR"	1
"VA Medical Center -Detroit"	2
"VA Outpatient Clinic -Mare Island"	1
"VAMC—Westside"	1
"YMCA East Belleville Center; YMCA Membership; YMCA annual fee"	1
"YMCA Memebership"	1
"yoga classes"	1

Goods and Services Provided	Frequency
Residential Adaption and Repair	
"(317) Independent Living Residence Adaptation 645"	2
"(317) Independent Living Residence Adaptation 645, Residential adaptations to allow a veteran to complete ILP."	1
"A&E services for home modification per ILP"	1
"Basic construction as approved on IL plan"	1
"Ch 31 One Time Miscellaneous Items Purchase—Reconstruction of front porch per IL plan"	1
"Gould's Discount Medical — Home Improvements"	1
"Herrera Engineering; house modifications; special contractual services"	1
"Home Mod Eval"	1
"Home Reab Equipment — Supply and set up bath mods (up)"	1
"Home Rehab Equipment — custom railing"	1
"Home modification: Railing for steps"	1
"Home safety evaluation"	1
"Kohler & Lentz Construction; Home modifications for IL case"	1
"Labor for installing shower grab bar and locksets"	1
"Lumber for ramp construction"	1
"Mobile Home Stuff Store, Inc; Plumbing repairs: complete water supply replumbing"	1
"Plans for modification"	1
"Provide & install toilet area grab bars w/fasteners"	1
"Provide and insall shower grab bar w/fasteners"	1
"Stair railing"	1
"Veterans Assistance Network; wood handrails; 18 in grab bars; installation grab bar"	1
"buyrailings.com; stair railing w/brackets"	1
"ramp installation"	1
"set up and instruct on stair glides"	1
set up and supply bath mods	1
"threshold Ramp"	1
"scaffolding"	1
"smoke detectors/fire extinguisher/co2 detector"	1
Education and Training	
"Computer Instruction 13"	1
"Driving Lessons"	1
IHL Institute of Higher Learning	1
"IHL Institutions of Higher Learning"	38
"IHL Institutions of Higher Learning – for period 2/5/08-7/23/08"	1
"IHL Institutions of Higher Learning; 24 training session"	1
"IHL Institutions of Higher Learning (College books)"	1
"IHL Institutions of Higher Learning; Central Community College-Hastings Degree"	1
"Individual/Independent Instruction / Trg 164"	1

(Continued)

Goods and Services Provided	Frequency
Jewish Vocational Services; non college degree	4
"Kendall & Davis, Inc.; computer training"	1
"Mastering MS Office Made Easy (CD-ROM version)"	1
"NCD Non-College Degree"	10
"OJT On the Job Training/Apprenticeship"	5
"PC Training 02/08-04/08"	1
"Solano County Community College"	1
"Training"	2
"Tutorial services 182"	1
"University of Alaska, Fall Term"	2
"Computer Instruction 13"	1
"Computer Training 11/8/07-2/1/08"	1
computer training	8
"1-year audio book subscription (2 CDs/month)"	1
"2 computer innstruction books"	1
Assistive Devices and Technology	
"Adapter"	1
"Adapter/converter"	1
"All Temperature system; IL-Heating System"	1
"Amplified phone with 911 pendent"	1
"Audio Equipment and Software"	1
"CPI*Contour living web; wedge cushions/with massage; shipping charge"	1
"Cap Tel phone for hearing impaired"	1
"Ch 31 non-Contractual Special . . . \r\n"	1
Computer Evaluation Services 21, Technical evaluation for computer hardware and software needs.	2
"Computer installation"	1
"Computer repair"	1
"Exercycle"	1
"Forced Heater"	1
"GPS System"	1
"Installation of Camera Security System"	1
"KID 1240 talking dictionary with headphones"	1
"Kendall & Davis; notebook computer"	1
"King size adjustable bed with massage"	1
"Lift chair with heat and massage"	1
"Metal Detection Club Mem. 1 yr,"	1
"Pride GL 358M lift chair w/set up and delivery"	1
"Quick 2008 software"	1
"Security system per IILP"	1
"Sleep number bed w/ frame"	1

Goods and Services Provided	Frequency
"Solutions4Sure - HP IPAQ"	1
"Spinlife -hoyer hyrdaulic patient lifter"	1
"Sports authority; Treadmill, delivery & assembly, 4 yr warranty"	1
"Surge protector"	1
"True Freedom Mobility; Lift chair"	1
"US Computers Inc; Shipping/handling fees for computer and furnitures"	1
"Washer"	1
"Wireless router"	1
"day Timer Smartech"	1
"massagin seat cushion"	1
"set and instruct on 4 wheel scooter"	1
"set and instruct on scooter lift with swing arm."	1
"set and instruction for lift chair."	1
"speakers"	1
"washer/dryer"	1
"Electric Jar Opener"	1
Adaptive Equipment	
"All in one accessibility -adaptive equipment"	1
"24-Inch Grab Bar for Commode"	1
"ALI*AMIMED INC.; Backrest air obusforme grey; shipping charge"	1
"Alex Orthopedic; Walking Cane; Shipping charge"	1
"Appointment book"	1
"Automobile seat cushion"	1
"Big-Handle Cup"	1
"Bowl, blue"	1
"COLDERS, INC.; Bed & Chair -Independent Living"	1
"Chair"	2
"Colder's; TempurPedic King Size Solution Mattress and Box Sp; HTC-1650 Massage Chair"	1
"Computer chair"	1
"Deluxe swivel seat cushion, UpEasy lifting cushion seat assist (plus shipping)"	1
"Dry Erase Board & Calendar"	1
"E-Pill 7-day organizer/reminder sys"	1
"Elastic Shoelaces"	1
"Ergonomic Office & Shop Stool"	1
"Eyemasters; eye glasses"	1
"Frame, Lenses"	1
"Gallon Tipper"	1
"Glide rail & shower wand,PT-WR28R,LABOR"	1
"Grab bar specialists, Inc.; handi-grip portable grab bar and shipping"	1
"Handicap aid equipment"	1
"IL Adaptive Equipment \r\nCh 31 Special Equipment"	1

(Continued)

Goods and Services Provided	Frequency
"IL Adaptive equipment, Shipping and Handling\r\nCh 31 Special Equipment"	1
"Kitchen Cart w/3 Shelves and Casters"	1
"Lamp for independent living and surge protector"	1
"MAXIAUDS; CO2 Alarm; shiping charge"	1
"Medication dispenser, phone, printer, mouse"	1
"Mother Earth Design INC.; Trigger point pillow; shipping charge"	1
"Office furniture"	1
"Ontime supplies; ergonomic chair, dry erase board"	1
"Organizing service"	1
"Perching Stool, Height Adjustable, 250lb Capacity"	1
"Pill Container AM PM"	1
"Pill box with alarm, grab bars"	1
"Portable Lift Cushion, 250 1b Capacity"	1
"ProMED; Tempurpedic bed"	1
"ProMed; Long-handled bath brush"	1
"Queen Matt, Box, Tempura Symphony pillow"	1
"Queen mattress"	1
"Rehab Engineering Inc.; Large Handle cups; walker, 3-inch wheels,	1
300lbs. capacity; 24-inch grab bar, inside tub"	
"Rolling laundry cart & ergonomic grabber"	1
"SENIORSHOPS.COM; Safety bed rail"	1
"Sit/Stand Stool"	1
"Sliding Shelves (for Bathroom Cabinet)"	1
"Small Stool"	1
"Sock/Stocking Aid"	1
"Special equipment — one-handed jar opener, suction cup plates, suction cup bowls"	1
"Stocking Aid w/Loops"	1
"Stool"	1
"Trio Jar and Bottle Opener"	1
"Tub safety bar and lever door handles (QTY 6)"	1
"Universal Opener"	1
"Vocational Resource Services; good grips eating utensils; sock assist; elastic shoelaces"	1
"Vocational Resource Services; locking elevated toilet seat w/ arms; special equipment"	1
"Walker Furniture; mattress, frame and bed cover"	1
"adaptive aids"	1
"computer desk"	1
"desk and chair"	1

Goods and Services Provided	Frequency
"desk chair"	1
"grab bar"	1
"laundry cart"	1
"non Skid Mat"	1
"rolling stool with s/h"	1
"set up and instruct for K adj bed."	1
sock aid	1
"www.themedicalclub.com; HC-SP-S 1119 Super pole and shipping"	1
Computer and Camera Equipment	
"Adaptive computer system"	1
"Adobe Photoshop"	1
"Camera, case, warranty, & Adobe Elements"	1
"Camera, fash card, carea kit"	1
"Camera, memory card"	1
"Camera/Peripherals"	1
"Carrying case (for laptop) & surge protector"	1
"Computer"	1
"Computer & peripherals"	1
"Computer ILLP"	2
"Computer Masters; Computer System (IL)"	1
"Computer Set up-Intenet"	1
"Computer System, desk & chair"	1
"Computer and printer and accessories"	1
"Computer hardware/software and computer desk/chair"	1
"Computer speakers"	1
"Computer system with 19 inch moniter, printer software"	1
"Computer, Printer, Monitor, and Web Cam"	1
"Computer, flash, microsoft office pro 07"	1
"Computer/Printer/Accessories/Recliner/Computer cha"	1
"Computer/Printer/Peripherals"	3
"Dell -desktop, surge protector, and printer"	1
"Dell Desk top computer"	1
"Dell Laptop computer package"	1
"Dell all in one printer"	1
"Dell computer, Printer, surge protector"	1
"Dell; monitor and desktop"	1
"Desktop computer system"	1
"Digital Camera"	1
"Epson Photo inkjet printer"	1
"Flash Drive"	2
"IILP -Computer equipment"	1
"IILP -Digital Photography Equipment"	1
"Internet Service"	1

(Continued)

Goods and Services Provided	Frequency
"Internet fees and wireless card"	1
"Journey Ed; PhotShop CS4"	1
"Laptop and Accessories"	1
"Laptop computer"	1
"Laptop computer system, 3-year warranty"	1
"Laptop, case,surge prot, flash drive"	1
"MS Office Home and Student 2007"	1
"Microsoft Office Proffessional Upgrade Software"	1
"Milwaukee PC -75; Laptop computer system"	1
"Nikon Coolpix Digital Camera"	1
"Nikon Speedlight Flash for digital camera"	1
"Norton AntiVirus 2008"	1
"Office Depot; PC"	1
"PC"	1
"Printer"	1
"Staples; computer and accessories"	1
"Staples; computer assories"	1
"Toshiba laptop computer system"	1
"US Computers Inc; desktop computer system; monitor 19 in LCD; HP printer all-in-one"	1
"Video Camcorder kit"	1
"XPS One, Red—Dell Desk Top computer"	1
"adapted computer"	1
"all in one printer"	1
"cable for computer purchased"	1
"computer"	4
"computer printer/cables"	1
"computer w/19 inch monitor, 4n1 printer + internet"	1
"computer, printer"	1
"computer, printer, associated supplies"	1
"desktop computer system"	1
"digital camera, case, warranty"	1
"laptop computer and printer"	1
"laptop printer"	1
"monitor, camera, headset"	1
"printer, cable, delivery"	1
"quicken and mavis"	1
"software-printer"	1
"usb cable and ink"	1
Avocational/Leisure Equipment	
"Elite Duo 1500 Workbench and excess weight charge"	1

Goods and Services Provided	Frequency
"Windward boats; glasspro boat, motor, trailer"	1
"10" table saw, delivery"	1
"12 inch dualbevel slide mitersaw 77-141-614 Bosc"	1
"2hp soft start fixed and plunge base router"	1
"6 Tool Cordless Combo Kit"	1
"Craftsman 10 inch table saw"	1
"Craftsman fixed base router/table combo"	1
"Embroidery Machine & Accessories, Classes"	1
"Jarvi Facetron; Facitron Machine with grit; shipping"	1
"Music Production Equipment"	2
"Rikon 18 inch bandsaw, excess weight charge"	1
"Rikon 6 inch jointer"	1
"Searrs; rts bit saw nailer plnr sander warrenties"	1
"Sears; router and table and warrenty"	1
"Shopsmith Mark V"	1
"Tracrac T3B portable miter saw sta Bosch"	1
"drill press, protection agreement, shipping"	1
"The Rock Shed; Thumlers tumbler; 5lbs 60/90 grit; 5lbs 120/220 grit"	1
"(IL books) Audio Books"	1
"8 Spools of Thread"	1
"Accessory Kit, Bench Clamp and shipping for workbench"	1
"Bagpipe Accessories"	1
"Bagpipe Uniform & Accessories"	1
"Blick Art -acrylic paint and supplies"	1
"Bosch Tool Kit"	1
"Cookbooks"	1
"Fishing equipment"	1
"Metal detector items"	1
"Models"	1
"Silversmithing and Engraving Tools/Equipment"	1
"Trailer hitch"	1
"Vibration reduction lens"	1
"Walmart; camping equipment"	1
"car rack"	1
Other Goods and Services	
"Ch 31 Books"	1
"Supplies"	1
"(1) Specialized Equipment Acquisition 589"	1
"3 year extended laptop warranty"	1
"3-month membership, Dickinson Parks & Recreation"	1
"3-month membership, West River Community Center"	1
Abilities Group	2
"Assistive Technological Services 599"	2

(Continued)

Goods and Services Provided	Frequency
"Center for Independent Living"	2
"Club T.E.A.M "	1
"Delivery"	1
"Downing Properties LLC "	1
"Equipment and Installtion Fee"	1
"Equipment for IL"	1
"IL Equipment"	1
"IL Supplies, Shipping and Handling\r\nCh 31 Special Equipment"	1
"IL equipment & ship"	1
"Installation ILLP"	1
"Maids PO#Julia 300; Tub rails; shipping charge"	1
"Membership"	1
"Merry Maids; maid services; fee, intial; Refrigerator cleaning"	1
"PROMED; IL Purchases"	1
"ProMED; IL Equipment"	1
"Service Charge"	1
"Set-up and Shipping (for exercycle)"	1
"Shipping and Handling"	1
"Shipping/delivery charges for CD-ROM"	1
"Independence Inc."	1
"VR&E/28 "	1
"Voc Rehab Panel, PO 348-08-039 dtd 7/23/08"	1
"Ship Boat to Molokai"	1
"warranty"	1
"Cub Cadet Bagger"	1
"Ariens Snowblower"	1
"Cub Cadet Riding Lawn Mower"	1
"McGavic Outdoot power equipment; lawn tractor and delivery"	1
"lawn tractor"	1
"one snowblower"	1

Source: GAO analysis of 182 case files of veterans entering the IL track during fiscal year 2008.

Appendix IV: Rehabilitation Rates by Regional Office, FY 2008 Independent Living Track Entrants

	Entrants with One IL Plan	Transfers to a VR&E Employment Track	Rehabilitated	Discontinued	Open	Rehabilitation Rate
National	2274	34	1987	122	131	89%
Muskogee	35	0	35	0	0	100%
Reno	13	1	12	0	0	100%
Togus	9	0	9	0	0	100%
Huntington	5	1	4	0	0	100%
Boise	4	0	4	0	0	100%
Wichita	3	1	2	0	0	100%
Roanoke	2	0	2	0	0	100%
Pittsburgh	2	0	2	0	0	100%
San Juan	2	0	2	0	0	100%
Manchester	2	0	2	0	0	100%
Montgomery	202	2	198	1	1	99%
Hartford	77	2	74	1	0	99%
Louisville	64	1	62	0	1	98%
Newark	59	0	58	0	1	98%
Atlanta	119	0	114	3	2	96%
Phoenix	141	0	135	6	0	96%
San Diego	41	1	38	1	1	95%
Nashville	18	0	17	0	1	94%
Denver[a]	66	0	62	3	1	94%
New York	161	1	149	10	1	93%
Waco	69	0	64	2	3	93%
Philadelphia	26	0	24	1	1	92%
Honolulu	37	0	34	3	0	92%
Milwaukee	20	0	18	1	1	90%
Seattle	29	1	25	3	0	89%
Salt Lake City	27	0	24	1	2	89%
Columbia	26	0	23	0	3	88%
Detroit	131	3	113	7	8	88%

(Continued)

	Entrants with One IL Plan	Transfers to a VR&E Employment Track	Rehabilitated	Discontinued	Open	Rehabilitation Rate
Houston	73	1	63	8	1	88%
Oakland	163	5	138	12	8	87%
Albuquerque	88	0	76	11	1	86%
Winston-Salem	22	0	19	2	1	86%
St. Paul	7	0	6	1	1	86%
Baltimore	7	0	6	0	0	86%
Indianapolis	79	4	64	4	7	85%
St. Louis	24	1	19	2	2	83%
Buffalo	20	0	16	0	4	80%
Portland	20	1	15	2	2	79%
St. Petersburg	116	1	90	4	21	78%
Sioux Falls	9	0	7	0	2	78%
Fort Harrison	4	0	3	1	0	75%
Boston	4	0	3	1	0	75%
Los Angeles	97	5	67	9	16	73%
Providence	18	0	13	1	4	72%
Jackson	7	0	5	1	1	71%
Anchorage	7	1	4	0	2	67%
Little Rock	26	1	16	4	5	64%
Lincoln	16	0	10	4	2	63%
Fargo	8	0	5	2	1	63%
Des Moines	21	0	13	2	6	62%
New Orleans	7	0	4	1	2	57%
Chicago	4	0	2	2	0	50%
Cleveland	35	0	17	4	14	49%
Washington[b]	2	0	0	1	1	0%
White River Junction	0	0	0	0	0	n.a.
Wilmington	0	0	0	0	0	n.a.

Source: GAO analysis of VA data. [a] The Denver Regional Office includes totals for the Cheyenne, Wyoming office. This office is considered a satellite office of Denver.

[b] The Washington Regional Office, located in the District of Columbia, was renamed the National Capital Region Benefits Office in November 2012.

Note: This table represents those veterans with only one IL plan who entered the IL track in fiscal year 2008 and who were rehabilitated by the end of fiscal year 2011. We calculated the IL rehabilitation rate using open IL cases, as well as those cases that were closed by VR&E as "rehabilitated" or "discontinued." We did not include IL track veterans who were transferred to another VR&E employment track. VR&E calculates the IL rehabilitation rate using only closed cases.

APPENDIX V: DAYS TO COMPLETE INDEPENDENT LIVING PLANS, VETERANS ENTERING THE INDEPENDENT LIVING TRACK DURING FY 2008

Regional Office	Number of veterans completing their IL plan	Minimum	Mean	Median	Maximum
Roanoke	2	888	895	895	906
Buffalo	16	263	676	771	1,151
Des Moines	13	142	621	657	1,147
Chicago	2	413	621	621	829
Denver[a]	62	0	581	628	931
Sioux Falls	7	183	581	449	1,026
New Orleans	4	168	581	614	924
Los Angeles	67	110	577	566	1,289
St. Petersburg	90	102	552	522	1,121
Seattle	25	150	548	533	1,180
Jackson	5	278	533	405	913
Portland	15	194	526	511	1,209
Cleveland	17	0	515	343	1,154
San Juan	2	343	500	500	657
Togus	9	223	486	310	1,114
Columbia	23	110	482	321	1,172
Honolulu	34	18	457	508	1,052
Oakland	138	55	453	457	917
Detroit	113	0	446	416	975
Indianapolis	64	4	446	416	1,304
Lincoln	10	0	446	555	793
Anchorage	4	131	442	497	646
Milwaukee	18	66	431	398	909
Houston	63	22	420	358	1,129
Boise	4	66	409	274	1,030
Providence	13	4	398	303	986

(Continued)

Regional Office	Number of veterans completing their IL plan	Minimum	Mean	Median	Maximum
Philadelphia	24	4	380	387	796
Salt Lake City	24	7	380	325	906
Muskogee	35	40	369	292	1,085
Fargo	5	0	369	321	738
Nashville	17	128	365	321	836
Winston-Salem	19	0	362	300	1,264
Manchester	2	340	362	362	387
Baltimore	6	0	358	435	771
Wichita	2	124	358	358	592
Atlanta	114	69	351	292	1,103
New York	149	22	340	336	942
Hartford	74	0	329	307	836
Little Rock	16	80	325	208	763
Pittsburgh	2	215	318	318	416
Albuquerque	76	37	310	270	891
Waco	64	84	310	256	1,249
Fort Harrison	3	194	310	292	446
San Diego	38	153	307	292	544
Newark	58	26	300	248	829
Louisville	62	44	296	219	891
St. Louis	19	55	296	172	1,147
Phoenix	135	51	289	252	731
Huntington	4	47	267	270	475
Montgomery	198	44	234	208	1,085
Boston	3	91	226	278	307
Reno	12	80	205	186	446
St. Paul	6	0	150	99	329

Source: GAO analysis of VA data.

[a] The Denver Regional Office includes totals for the Cheyenne, Wyoming office. This office is considered a satellite office of Denver.

Note: This table represents those veterans with only one IL plan who entered the IL track during fiscal year 2008 and were rehabilitated by the end of fiscal year 2011. The White River Junction and Wilmington regional offices had no IL track entrants during fiscal year 2008. The Washington Regional Office, renamed the National Capital Region Benefits Office in November 2012, had two entrants during fiscal year 2008, but neither were rehabilitated by the end of fiscal year 2011.

Appendix VI: Independent Living Track Caseload Nationwide and by Regional Office, FY 2008-2011

Number of Veterans Who Entered the IL Track by Region Office, FY 2008-2011					
	Overall IL Entrant Count 2008-2011	**2008**	**2009**	**2010**	**2011**
NATIONAL	**9215**	**2465**	**2260**	**2209**	**2281**
Montgomery	908	215	264	189	240
Detroit	709	148	172	202	187
New York	702	178	177	179	168
Atlanta	627	128	99	204	196
St. Petersburg	523	121	104	146	152
Houston	471	82	138	113	138
Oakland	462	181	118	86	77
Phoenix	440	147	114	93	86
Indianapolis	360	93	71	116	80
Waco	264	74	61	52	77
Newark	259	68	62	68	61
Los Angeles	251	101	72	41	37
Hartford	231	82	56	53	40
Albuquerque	221	95	47	32	47
Cleveland	181	36	55	25	65
St. Louis	166	27	40	41	58
Louisville	164	66	50	32	16
Buffalo	154	24	25	54	51
Denver[a]	146	68	25	37	16
San Diego	144	41	47	25	31
Columbia	126	27	32	34	33
Muskogee	118	35	17	29	37
Des Moines	97	25	42	10	20
Honolulu	93	38	13	24	18
Reno	89	13	7	32	37
Jackson	85	7	27	27	24
Philadelphia	82	28	21	15	18
Little Rock	80	33	15	20	12
Seattle	79	30	25	10	14
Nashville	78	20	17	20	21
New Orleans	74	10	12	15	37
Winston-Salem	66	25	18	13	10
Salt Lake City	63	28	16	14	5
Huntington	58	6	8	20	24

(Continued)

Number of Veterans Who Entered the IL Track by Region Office, FY 2008-2011					
	Overall IL Entrant Count 2008-2011	2008	2009	2010	2011
NATIONAL	9215	2465	2260	2209	2281
Togus	58	9	19	10	20
Providence	58	19	16	17	6
Lincoln	58	18	35	5	0
Portland	56	22	10	7	17
Sioux Falls	46	11	22	6	7
Fargo	45	8	19	11	7
Baltimore	41	7	14	14	6
Milwaukee	38	20	6	6	6
St. Paul	31	9	12	7	3
Chicago	26	7	10	4	5
Fort Harrison	25	4	9	3	9
Roanoke	25	2	4	10	9
Boise	24	4	2	14	4
Pittsburgh	22	2	3	4	13
Washington[b]	22	4	2	4	12
Wichita	18	3	0	4	11
Anchorage	12	8	1	1	2
White River Junction	11	0	3	5	3
San Juan	9	2	0	3	4
Boston	8	4	3	1	0
Manchester	7	2	2	1	2
Wilmington	4	0	1	1	2

Source: GAO's analysis of VA administrative data.

[a] The IL entrant total for the Denver Regional Office includes the total number of veterans who entered the Cheyenne, Wyoming, office. This office is considered a satellite office of Denver.

[b] The Washington Regional Office, located in the District of Columbia, was renamed the National Capital Region Benefits Office in November 2012.

End Notes

[1] VA officials told us that the Washington Regional Office, located in the District of Columbia, was recently designated the "National Capital Region Benefits Office" in November 2012. For the purposes of our review, we will refer to this office as one of VA's regional offices.

The Manila Regional Office in the Philippines was not included in our review because it does not administer the IL track.

[2] To assess the reliability of these data, we interviewed knowledgeable officials and performed electronic tests to identify missing or erroneous data. We determined the data to be sufficiently reliable for our purpose, unless otherwise noted.

[3] Our review of IL track administration did not include reviewing the quality of internal or external assessments the VR&E program uses to determine the suitability of veterans for employment or the extent to which veterans' activities of daily living may be limited.

[4] Although not officially admitted into the IL track, veterans in VR&E's other tracks can receive IL services that may assist them in meeting their rehabilitation goals.

[5] Under 38 U.S.C. § 3120(d), a veteran's IL program "shall consist of such services…as the Secretary determines necessary to enable such veteran to achieve maximum independence in daily living."

[6] ADLs are basic activities that individuals perform on a daily basis, such as bathing, feeding, and dressing themselves.

[7] According to VA officials, IL services that "support emotional needs and/or avocational and leisure interests may be included in IL plans only when gains in independence are an anticipated result."

[8] The Veterans' Benefits Act of 2010 increased the cap to 2,700 effective "with respect to fiscal years beginning after the date of enactment of this Act." Pub. L. No. 111-275, § 801, 124 Stat. 2864, 2888. Because the enactment date of the Act was October 13, 2010 (fiscal year 2011), the cap of 2,700 veterans would have become effective starting in fiscal year 2012.

[9] 38 U.S.C. § 3102(a)(1)(A)(i) and (B). The law defines an employment handicap as an impairment, resulting in substantial part from a service-connected disability of a veteran's ability to prepare for, obtain, or retain employment consistent with the veteran's abilities, aptitudes, and interests. 38 U.S.C. § 3101(1). Veterans with a 10 percent service-connected disability may also be eligible to receive VR&E services, but not independent living services, if they have a serious employment handicap, which is defined as a significant impairment, resulting in substantial part from a service-connected disability rated at 10 percent or more, of a veteran's ability to prepare for, obtain or retain employment consistent with his or her abilities, aptitudes and interests. 38 U.S.C. §§ 3102(a)(2), 3101(7) and 3120(b). Moreover, servicemembers with a severe injury or illness are entitled to certain VR&E services, including independent living services. Pub. L. No. 110-181, § 1631(b), 122 Stat 3, 458 (2008), as extended by Pub. L. No. 112-56, § 231, 125 Stat. 711, 719 (2011)

[10] For veterans rated at 10 percent and veterans beyond their 12-year basic period of eligibility, the finding of a serious employment handicap is necessary to establish entitlement to VR&E services.

[11] 38 U.S.C. §§ 3102 and 3120(b).

[12] While VR&E's Central Office oversees regional offices that administer the IL track, it does not have direct line authority over regional staff. VBA's Office of Field Operations maintains this responsibility.

[13] VR&E has two performance measures for its IL rehabilitation rate. VR&E's fiscal year 2011 IL rehabilitation target was 92 percent, and its strategic target (or long-term goal) was 95 percent.

[14] VRCs work directly with veterans participating in all of VR&E's five tracks, not just the IL track.

[15] An employment-related plan is developed for veterans who are admitted to one of VR&E's other four tracks.

[16] 38 U.S.C. § 3105(d), 38 C.F.R. § 21.76(b). An additional period of 6 months is allowed if it would enable veterans to substantially increase their level of independence in daily living. In addition, VR&E may extend the duration up to 36 months for veterans with severe disabilities who served on active duty after September 11, 2001. 38 U.S.C. § 3105(d)(2)(A)(ii) and Department of Veterans Affairs, Veterans Benefits Administration,

Extension of Independent Living Services related to the Veterans Benefits Improvement Act of 2008 (Public Law 110-389), VR&E Letter 28-09-10 (January 30, 2009).

[17] Specific criteria must be met before approving new plans for IL services. These criteria include meeting requirements for participation in a program of IL services, and the worsening of the veteran's condition or other changes in the veteran's circumstances resulting in a substantial loss of independence. 38 C.F.R. § 21.284(b).

[18] VBA's Loan Guaranty Program administers two grants—the Specially Adapted Housing (SAH) grant and Special Housing Adaptation (SHA) grant—to help address the housing needs of veterans with service-connected disabilities.

[19] To receive medical devices and equipment through PSAS, VRCs must submit a service request to the veterans' VHA primary care physician. If the primary physician concurs with the VRC's request, he or she will submit a referral to PSAS to meet the veterans' needs.

[20] 38 C.F.R. § 21.283(e).

[21] VA pays monthly disability compensation to veterans with service-connected disabilities—injuries or diseases incurred or aggravated while on active military duty—according to the severity of the disability. VA's ratings are awarded in 10 percent increments, from 0 to 100 percent. Veterans with multiple disabilities receive a single composite (or combined) rating.

[22] Veterans of any age determined to be "unemployable" because of a combined service-connected disability rating between 60 and 90 percent, can qualify for an increase in their disability compensation to the amount paid to veterans with a combined service-connected disability rating of 100 percent.

[23] VR&E's policy states that the agency does not have the authority to purchase or rent automobiles, trucks, or other similar "conveyances" for veterans. Also, while VR&E may provide mobility aids such as wheelchairs to veterans, tractors or mowers should never be approved as a mobility aid. See Department of Veterans Affairs, Veterans Benefits Administration, *Purchase of Vehicles for Vocational Rehabilitation & Employment (VR&E) Participants under 38 U.S.C. Chapter 31 is prohibited*, VR&E Letter 28-13-08 (November 6, 2012).

[24] See appendix I for more information on the limits of our case file review.

[25] For confidence intervals for these estimates, see appendix I.

[26] The median cost per IL track case that year was about $3,900. At the 95 percent confidence interval, the amount of median expenditures per veteran who started an IL track case in fiscal year 2008 falls between $3,071 and $4,452. For additional confidence intervals for these estimates, see appendix I.

[27] VR&E officials told us that the law does not limit the number of IL plans VR&E can develop for a veteran, and as a result, veterans can have more than one plan. For our analysis, we included veterans who began only one plan during fiscal year 2008. Of the 2,465 veterans who began an IL plan during fiscal year 2008, 2,274—about 92 percent—had only one IL plan. In addition, our analysis excludes 34 veterans who entered the IL track during fiscal year 2008 but whose cases were subsequently transferred to another one of VR&E's employment tracks. We found that less than 1 percent of IL cases transferred to one of VR&E's employment tracks. See appendix I for more information about our analyses.

[28] We calculated this rate based on both closed and open IL cases for veterans beginning the IL track during fiscal year 2008. In our calculation of the IL rehabilitation rate, we did not include IL track veterans who were transferred to another VR&E employment track. In contrast, VR&E calculates its IL rehabilitation rate using only those IL cases that were closed as "rehabilitated" or "discontinued" during a fiscal year.

[29] In the Washington D.C. Regional Office, which VA now refers to as the National Capital Region Benefits Office, two veterans entered the IL track during fiscal year 2008. One case was discontinued, and one case was open at the end of fiscal year 2011.

[30] Twenty-six regional offices had more than 25 veterans enter the IL track during fiscal year 2008, while 30 offices had 25 or fewer veterans enter the IL track during the same time period. Two offices had no IL track entrants that year.

[31] Our analysis of the amount of time to rehabilitate IL participants is based on the 2,274 veterans who had a single IL plan developed in fiscal year 2008. These veterans represent about 92 percent of the total 2,465 veterans entering the IL track in fiscal year 2008.

[32] The St. Paul Regional Office had nine veterans enter the IL track during fiscal year 2008, while the Roanoke Regional Office had two veterans enter that year.

[33] We reported the average time to complete IL plans for 53 of VA's 56 regional offices because two offices did not have veterans begin the IL track in fiscal year 2008. Another office had two IL track veterans begin during this period, but these veterans were not "rehabilitated."

[34] While there was no clear pattern for the time it took veterans to complete their IL plans based on veterans' combined service-connected disabilities, totally disabled veterans took about a month longer on average to complete their IL plans than non-totally disabled veterans.

[35] Our model is based on the experiences of veterans who entered the IL track during fiscal years 2008 through 2011 and had only one IL plan during this time period. We used our model to estimate the probability of a veteran being rehabilitated within 2 years if the IL plan was begun at a regional office that had at least 50 IL cases during fiscal years 2008 through 2011.

[36] In general, programs of independent living may not exceed 24 months except under certain circumstances. An additional 6 months is allowed if it would enable veterans to substantially increase their level of independence in daily living. In addition, VR&E officials stated that they may extend the duration up to 36 months for veterans with severe disabilities who served on active duty on or after September 11, 2001.

[37] Our model shows that VR&E's rehabilitation rate increases by 4.3 percent for each additional 100 cases a regional office completes. The margin of error associated with these estimates ranged from 3.3 to 5.4 percent at the 95 percent confidence level.

[38] VR&E's policy manual states that contact via telephone, email, or mail can be used as alternatives when necessary. Department of Veterans Affairs, Vocational Rehabilitation and Employment, *Chapter 9: Guidelines for the Administration of An Independent Living Plan,* VR&E manual, Part IV, Section C, Chapter 9.

[39] VR&E's Quality Assurance (QA) Program at the national level periodically performs file reviews and site visits of selected regional offices to assess service delivery and compliance with VA regulations, procedures, and other directives. After the QA review or site visit, a report is provided to the regional office under review that summarizes the key results and findings.

[40] According to officials, the monthly in-person meeting requirement is only for the IL track, not VR&E's other employment-related tracks.

[41] VRCs we interviewed during our site visits reported relatively few challenges coordinating with SAH because not many IL cases are referred to this program for home modifications. In particular, we found in the 182 IL cases we reviewed that less than 3 percent were referred to SAH. VRCs commented that many veterans do not qualify for the SAH's home modification grants because of their eligibility requirements.

[42] 38 C.F.R § 21.216(b).

[43] Department of Veterans Affairs, Veterans Health Administration, VHA Directive 2010-022, *Vocational Rehabilitation: Chapter 31 Benefits, Timely Access to Health Care Services* (May 14, 2010).

[44] United States Department of Veterans Affairs, *Vocational Rehabilitation & Employment Services: Independent Living Participant Study* (September 26, 2008).

[45] VA Vocational Rehabilitation and Employment Task Force. *Report to the Secretary of Veterans Affairs: The Vocational Rehabilitation and Employment Program for the 21st Century Veteran* (2004).

[46] The standards for internal control in the federal government state that it is important for federal agencies to have timely information to help ensure efficient and consistent program administration. In addition, it is also critical for federal agencies, including those with highly decentralized program operations, to comprehensively identify risks that may impede

their ability to achieve program goals. See GAO, *Internal Control Management and Evaluation Tool,* GAO-01-1008G (Washington, D.C.: August 2001).

[47] VA is also mandated by Congress to conduct a longitudinal study of individuals in VR&E's programs, including the IL track, to determine the long-term outcomes of program participants. Results from this study are required to be reported to the House and Senate Veterans' Affairs Committees on an annual basis. Veterans' Benefits Improvement Act of 2008, Pub. L. No. 110-389, § 334, 122 Stat. 4145, 4172.

[48] United States Department of Veterans Affairs, Vocational Rehabilitation & Employment Services: Independent Living Participant Study (September 26, 2008).

[49] GAO-01-1008G .

[50] VR&E's guidelines for the administration of an independent living plan state that VRCs are required to obtain appropriate approval if IL costs exceed $25,000—not that all IL costs are required to be approved. See Department of Veterans Affairs, Vocational Rehabilitation and Employment, *Chapter 9: Guidelines for the Administration of An Independent Living Plan,* VR&E manual, M28, Part IV, Subpart iv, Chapter 9 (December 29, 2006). Furthermore, a 2010 VR&E policy letter outlines information that must be submitted by VRCs to obtain regional or Central Office approval of construction costs that exceed certain thresholds. However, this letter does not outline the requirements for non-construction related costs. Veterans Benefits Administration, *Review of Requests for Independent Living (IL) Construction Costs in Excess of $2,000,* VR&E Letter 28-11-05 (December 3, 2010).

[51] In 2008, the provision of riding lawn mowers was not specifically prohibited by VR&E policy.

[52] The case record indicates that the veteran was provided a boat to "significantly improve independent living and psychosocial functioning". At the time of assessment, the VRC noted that the veteran, who suffered from PTSD, was socially isolated but had an interest in fishing. However, the veteran's old boat "rotted away," and the cost for purchasing a new one was high. The VRC noted in the case file that because the veteran received a new boat, he was less depressed and his relationships with family and friends improved.

[53] VA's policy states that managerial cost accounting should be performed to measure and report the costs incurred by the agency. Specifically, each administration and its units should identify the cost of products and services provided. For example, in the case of a VHA medical center, the cost of a product or service may include a laboratory test, a medical ward bed, or a counseling session. The goal of this effort is to identify the product or service at the level in which it is rendered to an external customer, such as a veteran receiving benefits from a VA program. *Department of Veterans Affairs Managerial Cost Accounting: VA Financial Policies and Procedures,* volume III, chapter 3 (July 2010).

[54] According to these standards, managerial cost accounting is a fundamental part of an agency's financial management system, and each agency and its units should report the costs of their activities on a regular basis. This cost information can be used by Congress and federal executives in making decisions about allocating federal resources, authorizing and modifying programs, and evaluating performance. The cost information can also be used by program managers in making managerial decisions to improve operating economy and efficiency. Statement of Federal Financial Accounting Standards 4: *Managerial Cost Accounting Standards and Concepts..*

[55] GAO, *VA Vocational Rehabilitation and Employment: Better Incentives, Workforce Planning, and Performance Reporting Could Improve Program,* GAO-09-34 (Washington, D.C.: January 26, 2009).

[56] According to VR&E officials, some veterans in the IL track progress to a point where they may be able to pursue employment in one of VR&E's employment-related tracks; however, as noted earlier in this report, very few veterans make this transition—less than 1 percent of the 8,812 IL track veterans who had one plan during fiscal years 2008 through 2011.

[57] The standards for internal control emphasize the need to have controls over computerized information systems to ensure the data entered is complete and accurate (GAO-01-1008G). In addition, GAO's federal information system controls audit manual states that agencies

should establish procedures to provide reasonable assurance that all inputs into the application have been authorized, accepted for processing, and accounted for; and any missing or unaccounted for source documents or input files have been identified and investigated. GAO, *Federal Information System Controls Audit Manual (FISCAM),* GAO-09-232G (Washington, D.C.: February 2009).

[58] For confidence intervals for these estimates, see appendix I.

[59] 38 U.S.C. § 3120(e). According to agency officials, "IL plans" are the same as "programs" of independent living services and assistance.

[60] According to VR&E officials, entering "independent living case status" means that the veteran is admitted into the IL track. For more information on VR&E's policy, see Department of Veterans Affairs, Veterans Benefits Administration, *Increase in New Independent Living (IL) Programs Allowed by Congress*, VR&E Letter 28-11-06 (December 14, 2010).

[61] VR&E officials indicated that another IL plan may need to be developed to address subsequent needs that arise from a new medical condition or the progression of an existing one.

[62] "Operational" information could include the number of individual veterans being served. Furthermore, these standards state that all pertinent information should be identified, captured, and distributed in an efficient and timely manner. GAO, *Standards for Internal Control in the Federal Government,* GAO/AIMD-00-21.3.1 (Washington, D.C.: November 1999).

[63] Department of Veterans Affairs, Vocational Rehabilitation and Employment (VR&E) Case Management Portal Project, Version 1.0, Case Management Portal, Business Requirements Document (September 26, 2012).

[64] VR&E has used the CWINRS system since 2001 to track veteran cases through its process and to manage program costs. The "WINRS" part of the acronym represents the first 5 regional offices that tested the original system. These offices include Waco, Texas; Indianapolis, Indiana; Newark, New Jersey; Roanoke, Virginia; and Seattle, Washington.

[65] VR&E uses a "case status" approach to track veterans' movement through its process in the CWINRS system. Those veterans who are found eligible for IL benefits enter what VR&E refers to as the "IL Status" in the CWINRS system. Veterans officially enter this status once an IL plan has been agreed upon and approved by the veteran, counselor, and VR&E Officer

[66] We conducted pretests at the Washington, D.C. regional office and at VR&E headquarters to compare the information found in veterans' paper and electronic records. We found the electronic case records to be sufficient for our purpose. Certain cost information is required to be entered into CWINRS. Nonetheless, we did request a physical copy of the closure report for each veteran in our sample. These reports summarize veterans' participation in the IL track.

[67] Veterans in the IL track are considered by VR&E to be "rehabilitated" when either all goals of the IL plan have been achieved, or if not achieved, when (1) the veteran has attained substantial increase in the level of independence, (2) the veteran has maintained the increased level of independent for at least 60 days, and (3) further assistance is unlikely to significantly increase the veteran's level of independence. For veterans who are unable to successfully complete the IL track, their cases are entered into a "discontinued status" where they are closed. Veterans' cases that are still ongoing are classified as open.

[68] VA officials told us that Washington Regional Office, located in the District of Columbia, was recently designated the National Capital Region Benefits Office in November 2012. For the purpose of our review, we will refer to this office as one of VA's regional offices. Furthermore, our review of IL track administration did not include reviewing the quality of internal or external assessments the VR&E program uses to determine the suitability of veterans for employment or the extent to which veterans' activities of daily living may be limited.

[69] This group also excluded veterans who transferred to a VR&E employment track and veterans who had more than one instance of rehabilitation. Missing data on age and length of service further reduced our sample size to 8,655 veterans for modeling purposes.

[70] We defined partially disabled veterans as those having combined VA disability ratings of less than 100 percent. Fully disabled veterans had ratings of 100 percent.

[71] We linked each numeric disability code in our sample to one of 16 categories of disabilities defined by VA regulations.

[72] Schoenfeld residuals measure the difference between each observed covariate value for a failure at time *t* minus the expected value of the covariate. The expected value is taken over the probability distribution of failure probabilities at *t* for units in the risk set.

In: Veterans
Editor: Timothy C. Roberts
ISBN: 978-1-63117-046-1

Chapter 5

MILITARY FUNERAL HONORS AND MILITARY CEMETERIES: FREQUENTLY ASKED QUESTIONS*

Barbara Salazar Torreon

SUMMARY

This report is written in response to frequently asked questions about military funeral honors and military cemeteries. It provides information on the eligibility criteria, required components of the honor detail, and the funeral ceremony. It also cites legislation that mandates that the Department of Defense (DOD) make military funeral honors available to every eligible veteran upon request.

WHAT ARE MILITARY FUNERAL HONORS?

The Department of Defense (DOD) defines military funeral honors as the ceremonial paying of respect and the final demonstration of the country's gratitude to those who, in times of war and peace, have faithfully defended our

* This is an edited, reformatted and augmented version of a Congressional Research Service publication, CRS Report for Congress RS21545, prepared for Members and Committees of Congress, from www.crs.gov, dated May 3, 2013.

nation. Members of the funeral honors detail fold and present the American flag to the veteran's survivor and "Taps" is sounded.[1]

What Legislation Provides for the Implementation of the Current Military Funeral Honors Program?

The National Defense Authorization Act for FY2000, P.L. 106-65, as amended, sets out the requirements for funeral honors and mandates military honors at funerals for all eligible veterans.[2] The originating language can be found in the Strom Thurmond National Defense Authorization Act for Fiscal Year 1999, H.Rept. 105-736, Section 567: "The conferees agree that men and women, who have served honorably, whether in war or peace, deserve commemoration for their military service at the time of their death by an appropriate tribute. Burial honors are an important means of reminding Americans of the sacrifices endured to keep the Nation free."

What Agency Is Responsible for Administering the Military Funeral Honors Program?

The Department of Defense is responsible for providing military honors to eligible veterans. DOD Instruction 1300.15 updates policy and responsibilities for military funeral support. DOD has established a website that provides information including eligibility criteria, the text of relevant legislation, information for funeral directors, and related links, at https://www.dmdc.osd.mil/mfh/http://www.militaryfuneralhonors.osd.mil/. Questions or comments regarding the program can be addressed to: Deputy Assistant Secretary of Defense, (Military Community and Family Policy), 4000 Defense Pentagon, Room 5A726, Washington, DC 20380-400.

Who Is Eligible for Military Funeral Honors?

Military members in the following categories are eligible for military funeral honors: military personnel on active duty; former military members who served on active duty and were discharged under conditions other than dishonorable (as described below); members of the Selected Reserve; former members of the Selected Reserve who served at least one term of enlistment or period of initial obligated service and were discharged under conditions other than dishonorable; and former members of the Selected Reserve who were discharged due to a service-related disability.[3]

WHO IS INELIGIBLE FOR MILITARY FUNERAL HONORS?

Veterans are ineligible if convicted of a capital offense (as defined in the National Defense Authorization Act for FY2006, P.L. 109-163, Section 662), or when the circumstances involved would bring discredit upon the person's service or former service. Veterans are also ineligible if they were discharged from the military under dishonorable conditions. These conditions include dishonorable discharge, bad conduct discharge, dismissal from the service awarded by court-martial, other than honorable conditions discharge, and for officers who resign for the good of the service in lieu of courts-martial, which results in a discharge characterization of other than honorable conditions.

P.L. 109-163 (Section 662) modified titles 10 and 38 of the *U.S. Code*, to expand the prohibition against the interment of anyone in a national cemetery, as well as the use of military honors, for anyone convicted of a capital offense (as defined), or when the circumstances involved would bring discredit upon the person's service or former service. This language expands upon P.L. 105-116 that Congress passed in 1997. That law barred those convicted of capital crimes from being buried in a national cemetery. The 1997 law was ostensibly passed to prevent the possibility of Oklahoma City bomber Timothy McVeigh, a veteran, from being buried at Arlington National Cemetery. McVeigh was put to death on June 11, 2001.

Section 404 of P.L. 109-461 required the removal of Russell Wayne Wagner's remains from the columbarium at Arlington National Cemetery. An honorably discharged Vietnam veteran, Wagner was convicted of killing an elderly Maryland couple in 1994. Wagner died in 2005 while serving two life terms in prison. Because he was eligible for parole, he qualified for burial at Arlington. Following protests from the murdered couple's son, language was included in the Veterans Benefits, Health Care and Information Technology Act of 2006, P.L. 109-461, requiring the removal of Wagner's remains. The

Superintendent of the Arlington Cemetery reported that the cremated remains of Russell Wayne Wagner have been removed from Arlington National Cemetery and turned over to his sister.[4]

What Is the Required Composition of a Military Funeral Honors Detail?

The military services operate under service-specific policies; the honors vary from service to service and are dependent upon available resources. At the minimum, a funeral honors detail consists of two members of the Armed Forces, at least one of which is a member of the veteran's military service.

Funeral honors details may be augmented with volunteers who are military veterans and who are members of veterans' service organizations, such as the American Legion and the Veterans of Foreign Wars, or other appropriate organizations. The Authorized Provider Partnership Program (AP3) was established to provide training for these volunteers to standardize the quality of the honors rendered. Volunteers can participate as firing party members, pallbearers, and buglers, among other duties. When a trained bugler is not available, a recorded version of "Taps" may be played. DOD also approved the use of a ceremonial bugle, which contains a device in the bell of the bugle that plays a recorded version of "Taps." For more information, see the Department of Defense Ceremonial Bugle at https://www.dmdc.osd.mil/mfh/getLinks.do?tab=Bugle.

What Is the Protocol for the Flag Presentation to Next of Kin? 5 Are There Any Recent Changes?

After "Taps" has been played, the flag is folded into the tri-cornered shape. The folded flag is then presented to the next of kin or appropriate family member. Each branch of the Armed Forces uses its own wording for the presentation. Please note: A number of Internet postings have suggested that the flag presentation speech was changed from "On behalf of a grateful nation and the President of the United States" to "On behalf of a grateful nation and the Secretary of Defense." There is no new policy regarding the flag presentation. As stated below, each service has its own wording for the flag presentation:

U.S. Army—"This flag is presented on behalf of a grateful nation and the United States Army as a token of appreciation for your loved one's honorable and faithful service."

U.S. Navy—"On behalf of the President of the United States and the Chief of Naval Operations, please accept this flag as a symbol of our appreciation for your loved one's service to this Country and a grateful Navy."

U.S. Air Force—"On behalf of the President of the United States, the Department of the Air Force, and a grateful nation, we offer this flag for the faithful and dedicated service of rank and name of deceased."

U.S. Marine Corps—"On behalf of the President of the United States, the Commandant of the Marine Corps, and a grateful nation, please accept this flag as a symbol of our appreciation for your loved one's service to Country and Corps."

U.S. Coast Guard—"On behalf of the President of the United States, the Commandant of the Coast Guard, and a grateful nation, please accept this flag as a symbol of our appreciation for your loved one's service to Country and the Coast Guard."

Also, if the next of kin has expressed a religious preference or belief, "God bless you and this family, and God bless the United States of America" is added to the end of the statement.

How Many Military Funerals Requested Military Honors?

According to the Office of the Secretary of Defense (OSD) Legislative Affairs, in 2010, there were more than 236,000 military funerals requested. Of the 236,000 military funerals, 25,000 had an actual military bugler play "Taps," 15,000 had a bugler from a Veterans Service Organization (VSO) play "Taps," and 185,000 military funerals had ceremonial bugles.[6]

Are Military Bands Used at Military Funerals?

According to the historian at the Department of Veterans Affairs (VA) National Cemetery System (NCS), the use of military bands is extremely rare and the NCS does not maintain statistics on the use of military bands at military funerals.[7] The historian noted that even President Kennedy's funeral with full military honors at Arlington National Cemetery consisted of the 3rd Infantry's Colonial Fife and Drum Corps and not a military band.[8]

WHO IS RESPONSIBLE FOR MAKING THE ARRANGEMENTS FOR HONORS TO BE PERFORMED?

Honors are not performed automatically; they must be requested. Families of eligible veterans must request funeral honors through their funeral director. The funeral director is to contact the appropriate military service to arrange for the funeral honors detail. See the FAQs for Funeral Directors at https://www.dmdc.osd.mil/mfh/getLinks.do?tab=DirFAQ.

ARE MEMBERS OF THE MILITARY HONORS DETAIL PAID?

Members of the Ready Reserve[9] or retired military personnel who are part of a military funeral detail may receive pay, allowances, travel, and transportation reimbursements.[10] Ready Reserve personnel may also receive service credit for performing this duty.[11] Survivors are not charged for these services.

Section 571 of P.L. 107-314, the Bob Stump National Defense Authorization Act for FY2003, enacted December 2, 2002, provides for a flat rate daily stipend for members of the funeral honors detail who are not active duty military personnel. The current daily stipend is $50. The *U.S. Code* provides at 10 U.S.C. 1491(d) (1) that to support a funeral honors detail under this section, the Secretary of a military department may provide the following:

a) For a person who participates in a funeral honors detail (other than a person who is a member of the Armed Forces not in a retired status or an employee of the United States), either transportation (or reimbursement for transportation) and expenses or the daily stipend prescribed under paragraph (2).
b) For members of a veterans organization or other organization referred to in subsection (b) (2) and for members of the Armed Forces in a retired status, materiel, equipment, and training.

c) For members of a veterans organization or other organization referred to in subsection (b)(2), articles of clothing that, as determined by the Secretary concerned, are appropriate as a civilian uniform for persons participating in a funeral honors detail. Volunteers seeking reimbursement should complete DOD Standard Form 1164 and submit it to the unit with which they are volunteering.

How Many Military Funeral Honors for Veterans Requests Are Supported Only by Veterans Service Organizations?

DOD officials stated that the military, in accordance with the law, provides military personnel in every instance in which the eligible survivors have requested such honors. Defense officials note, however, that in some instances, funeral directors contact VSOs for such services with or without seeking military personnel assistance. It is not possible to know how often this occurs. Financial or other assistance (such as transportation, a stipend, or reimbursement for expenses) from the military for VSO services may be provided by a nearby military unit. This assistance comes from that unit's funds. In some instances, state governments have provided assistance or benefits to VSOs who perform these services.[12] For a list of current VSOs, see the *Directory 2012/2013, Veterans and Military Service Organizations State Directors of Veterans Affairs* at http://www.va.gov/vso/VSO-Directory_2012-2013.pdf.

What Military Honors Are Afforded to Individuals Interred or Inurned at Arlington National Cemetery?

Eligibility criteria for interment or inurnment can be obtained from the Arlington National Cemetery Website: http://www.arlingtoncemetery.mil/FuneralInformation/EstablishServices.aspx or from the Interment Services Branch at (703) 607-8585. Once eligibility is determined, honors are afforded according to rank. Enlisted personnel receive standard honors and a firing party. Commissioned and warrant officers receive standard honors, a firing party, and may request the caisson and escort troops. Those individuals who are eligible for inurnment in the columbarium receive the standard honors and a firing party. All may request a military chaplain to preside over the services. Effective January 1, 2009, all service members who die from wounds received as a result of enemy action and are being interred, inurned, or memorialized at Arlington National Cemetery are eligible to receive full military funeral honors. Additional details are in the *Administrative Guide to Information and Burial at Arlington National Cemetery* at http://www.arlingtoncemetery.mil/docs/FuneralInfo_AdminGuide 2InfoBurial_ANC.pdf and http:/ /www.arlingtoncemetery.mil/Funeral Infor mation/MilitaryHonors.aspx.

What Are the Available Emblems of Belief for Placement on Government Headstones and Markers?

A current list of the approved emblems of belief can be found on the U.S. Department of Veterans Affairs website at http://www.cem.va.gov/hmm/. An emblem of belief for Wicca, the pentacle, was added to the list in 2007.[13] According to the website, no graphics (logos, symbols, etc.) are permitted on government-furnished headstones or markers other than the approved emblems of belief, the Civil War Union Shield, the Civil War Confederate Southern Cross of Honor, and the Medal of Honor insignias. The graphics of 20 representative emblems of belief for placement on government-furnished headstones/markers is depicted on p.4 of the form "Claim for Standard Government Headstone or Marker for Placement in a Private Cemetery or a State Veterans' Cemetery" at http://www.va.gov/vaforms/va/pdf/VA40-1330.pdf.

Are Same-Sex Partners Allowed to be Buried at Arlington National Cemetery? What Other Funeral Benefits Are Allowed for Same-Sex Partners?

According to the DOD, same-sex partners are not allowed to be buried at Arlington or to receive other death benefits that military spouses currently receive. With the 2010 repeal by P.L. 111-321 of the "Don't Ask, Don't Tell" law, the DOD has extended some benefits to same-sex domestic partners of military members. However, the Defense of Marriage Act (DOMA) prohibits the DOD from making available other benefits now provided to heterosexual military spouses and their children, including death benefits. The DOMA is currently under review by the U.S. Supreme Court. For additional information, see former Secretary of Defense Leon Panetta's February 11, 2013 statement on the Extension of Benefits to Same-Sex Partners at http://www.defense.gov/releases/release.aspx?releaseid=15809 and the official DOD memorandum listing all the benefits for same-sex partners at http://www.defense.gov/news/SameSexBenefitsMemo.pdf.

End Notes

[1] Department of Defense Instruction 1300.15, "Military Funeral Support," October 22, 2007, at http://www.dtic.mil/ whs/directives/corres/pdf/130015p.pdf.

[2] 10 U.S.C. 1491.

[3] According to CRS Report RL30802, Reserve Component Personnel Issues: Questions and Answers, by Lawrence Kapp, "The Selected Reserve contains units and individuals most essential to wartime missions, in accordance with the national security strategy. They have priority over other reservists for training and equipment. Members of the Selected Reserve are generally required to perform one weekend of training each month ('inactive duty for training' or IDT, also known as 'weekend drill') and two weeks of training each year ('annual training' or AT, sometimes known colloquially as 'summer camp') for which they receive pay and benefits."

[4] Document available at http://www.arlingtoncemetery.net/rwwagner.htm.

[5] Military Funeral Honors Commander's Reference, Flag Presentation Protocol, Department of Defense at http://www.mfhcmdrs.osd.mil/mfhcr_edu_present.htm, and https://www.dmdc.osd.mil/mfh/getLinks.do?tab=Flag.

[6] Information provided to CRS by the Office of the Secretary of Defense (OSD) Legislative Affairs Office on July 7, 2011. Note: Current data is pending from DOD. These statistics will be updated as soon as the data is released.

[7] Information provide by Sarah Leach, historian with the VA's National Cemetery System, on July 7, 2011.

[8] The Last Salute: Civil and Military Funerals 1921-1969, Chapter 23, "President John F. Kennedy State Funeral 22-25 November 1963" at http://www.history.army.mil/books/Last_Salute/ch23.htm. For more information on military bands, see "Strike up the Band" by Mark Cantrell, Military Officer, October 2011, pp. 50-55.

[9] According to CRS Report RL30802, Reserve Component Personnel Issues: Questions and Answers, by Lawrence Kapp, "The Ready Reserve is the primary manpower pool of the reserve components. Members of the Ready Reserve will usually be called to active duty before members of the Standby Reserve or the Retired Reserve. The Ready Reserve is made up of the Selected Reserve, the Individual Ready Reserve, and the Inactive National Guard."

[10] 37 U.S.C. 435.

[11] 10 U.S.C. 12732(a) (2) (E).

[12] In consultation with David F. Burrelli, CRS specialist in National Defense, Foreign Affairs, Defense, and Trade Division on February 5, 2008. See also the Authorized Provider Partnership Program (AP3) website with a link to Standard Form 1164 "Claim for Reimbursement for Expenditures on Official Business" at https://www.dmdc.osd.mil/mfh/getLinks.do?tab=AP3.

[13] Settlement agreement and stipulation of dismissal in the case of Circle Sanctuary v. Nicholson, U.S. Dist. Ct., Western Dist. of Wisconsin, Case No. 06-C-0660-S.

INDEX

C

D

E

F

G

H

I

O

P

Q

R

U

V

W

X

Y